The Big Book of

Diabetic Desserts

Decadent and Delicious Recipes
Perfect for People with Diabetes

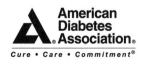
American Diabetes Association®
Cure • Care • Commitment®

Jackie Mills, MS, RD

Director, Book Publishing, Robert Anthony; *Managing Editor, Book Publishing,* Abe Ogden; *Editor,* Laurie Guffey; *Production Manager,* Melissa Sprott; *Composition,* American Diabetes Association; *Cover Design,* pixiedesign, llc; *Photography,* Taran Z, *Printer,* Transcontinental Printing.

Printed in Canada
1 3 5 7 9 10 8 6 4 2

The suggestions and information contained in this publication are generally consistent with the *Clinical Practice Recommendations* and other policies of the American Diabetes Association, but they do not represent the policy or position of the Association or any of its boards or committees. Reasonable steps have been taken to ensure the accuracy of the information presented. However, the American Diabetes Association cannot ensure the safety or efficacy of any product or service described in this publication. Individuals are advised to consult a physician or other appropriate health care professional before undertaking any diet or exercise program or taking any medication referred to in this publication. Professionals must use and apply their own professional judgment, experience, and training and should not rely solely on the information contained in this publication before prescribing any diet, exercise, or medication. The American Diabetes Association—its officers, directors, employees, volunteers, and members—assumes no responsibility or liability for personal or other injury, loss, or damage that may result from the suggestions or information in this publication.

♾ The paper in this publication meets the requirements of the ANSI Standard Z39.48-1992 (permanence of paper).

ADA titles may be purchased for business or promotional use or for special sales. To purchase more than 50 copies of this book at a discount, or for custom editions of this book with your logo, contact Lee Romano Sequeira, Special Sales & Promotions, at the address below, or at LRomano@diabetes.org or 703-299-2046.

For all other inquiries, please call 1-800-DIABETES.

American Diabetes Association
1701 North Beauregard Street
Alexandria, Virginia 22311

Library of Congress Cataloging-in-Publication Data

Mills, Jackie, 1961-
  The big book of diabetic desserts / Jackie Mills.
     p. cm.
  Includes index.
  ISBN 978-1-58040-274-3 (alk. paper)
  1. Diabetes—Diet therapy—Recipes. 2. Desserts. I. Title.
  RC662.M55 2007
  641.5'6314—dc22
                          2007018183

On the cover: Lemon–Spice Carrot Cake with Cream Cheese Frosting (see recipe, page 14)

This book is dedicated to
the loving memory of my parents,
Taylor and Creasie Mills.

Contents

Acknowledgements

Writing a cookbook is a group effort, and this one was made possible only because of the many generous people who supported and helped me along the way.

Thanks to Rob Anthony, who got the ball rolling and had the confidence that I could write a great dessert cookbook for people with diabetes.

Deepest gratitude to my sister Carol Lundy and my dear friends Dina Cheney, Judy Feagin, Jan Fitzpatrick, and Julia Rutland, who inspired and encouraged me even when my cookies crumbled.

Thanks to Joyce Hendley, Nancy Hughes, Dana Jacobi, and Robyn Webb, who gave me invaluable advice and answered hundreds of questions (I owe you all!).

Special appreciation to my agent, Beth Shepard, for her capable and intelligent guidance.

Thanks to Laurie Guffey for her editorial expertise, and to Lyn Wheeler for her exactitude in doing the nutrition analysis of the recipes.

And gratitude to all the fine people behind the scenes at the American Diabetes Association who work to prevent and cure diabetes and improve the lives of those affected by diabetes.

And finally, I give exceptional thanks to my husband, Nick Rutyna, for being the love of my life and for loading the dishwasher every night.

Introduction

ISN'T IT ALWAYS THE CASE that you crave more of what you're supposed to have less of? Using the recipes in this book, you can manage your menus to include the sweets you yearn for, yet stay within the carb and calorie targets of your eating plan.

The recipes found here are delicious compromises between often disappointing sugar-free, fat-free desserts and sugar-laden, high-calorie sweets that should only be a very rare treat. Most often these recipes use a combination of granulated sugar, brown sugar, honey, or molasses along with the granular no-calorie sweetener sucralose (Splenda®). Because most of the recipes use less sugar instead of no sugar, you'll find that the desserts are mouth-watering and enjoyable, but with carb counts that make it possible for them to fit into a balanced meal plan. Best of all, the portion sizes, though not super-sized, are large enough to please the hungriest sweet tooth.

You can and should enjoy desserts without feeling that you're having something second rate or that tastes "good for you." These desserts are so satisfying and delicious, you'll be happy to share them with others whether or not they are living with diabetes.

Budgeting for Brownies

If you are newly diagnosed with diabetes or you've lived with it for years, you undoubtedly know from your diabetes educator or dietitian how many grams of carb you should have each day.

Figuring out how to incorporate dessert into a healthy menu is a matter of simple math.

In controlling blood sugar levels, the number of grams of carb you eat or drink is more important than the source of the carb. (Although, for good nutrition, it always helps if the carb grams are from whole grains, vegetables, and fruits.) For example, if you would like a Cocoa Brownie (page 205) for lunch tomorrow, you can easily fit one into your carb budget. Let's say that your eating plan allows you to have 45 grams of carb at lunch and you're planning on a menu of a turkey sandwich and a small apple. The apple and two slices of whole wheat bread for the sandwich add up to about 45 grams of carb. But, if you make the sandwich open face, with only one slice of bread, you'll have about 15 carbs left—just enough to fit in a brownie. The carbs from desserts must be substituted for—not added to—the number of carbs allowed on your eating plan.

> "In controlling blood sugar levels, the number of grams of carb you eat or drink is more important than the source of the carb."

Of course, you can't give up eating nutrient and fiber-rich breads, grains, starchy vegetables, and fruits so that you can have a brownie at every meal! Moderation, variety, and calorie and fat budgeting are always important to ensure your health and well-being. Go ahead and treat yourself on occasion. Just know that desserts don't contain the vitamins, minerals, and fiber that grains and vegetables have, and in the majority of cases, sweets have more calories and fat than a grain or vegetable serving with the same amount of carbohydrate.

Because weight loss or weight control is a major goal for many people with diabetes, remember to budget not only carbs, but calories, too. Note the number of servings and the serving size listed with each recipe. Train your eye and your appetite that a 9-inch pie serves 8 people, not 4, and an ample serving of pudding is 1/2 cup, not 1 cup.

Here's one thing you don't have to think about with these yummy desserts: all of them are have less than 1.5 grams of saturated fat per serving and virtually no trans fat. People who have diabetes are more likely to have heart disease, and a major risk factor for heart disease is high blood cholesterol. Saturated fat and trans fat raise blood cholesterol and should be kept at an absolute minimum.

Oh, Sugar!

Sugar makes foods taste sweet. Everyone knows that, but sugar does so much more than add sweetness. These recipes were developed with just enough sugar to take advantage of the goodness it brings to desserts, but yet low enough in carbs that you can easily incorporate them into your eating plan. Because there's less sugar, though, there are some differences you will notice with these recipes.

Sugar caramelizes as it heats, which creates the desirable brown, tender crust on a cake or muffin that we all love so much. With low-sugar desserts, you'll find some browning, but not to the same degree as in traditional baked goods.

Sugar also acts as a preservative by helping to retain moisture in baked goods, so with less sugar, foods dry out and get stale faster. Plan on serving these desserts within a day or two of baking, or freeze them. You'll find storage recommendations with recipes where appropriate.

Cakes and quick breads made with less sugar don't rise as much as their high-sugar counterparts. Gluten is the protein in flour that creates tiny compartments that trap the gases formed by leavening agents (baking powder and/or baking soda). When less sugar is used, it allows the gluten that is formed to be stronger. The stronger the gluten, the more resistant it is to expansion from the gases, and the less a cake or muffin will rise. Also, with less sugar, the coagulation or "setting" of a batter takes place at lower temperature. So, the cake bakes faster and spends less time in the oven rising.

Sugar plays an important part in frozen desserts, too. In the homemade versions of ice cream and yogurt you'll find here (and also in commercial varieties), the ice crystals are larger than in high-sugar versions. Sugar holds some of the water in sweeter frozen desserts, which lowers the freezing point and makes the ice crystals smaller. Smaller ice crystals give a creamier texture. So low-sugar frozen desserts won't be as smooth and creamy as their high-sugar counterparts.

The Well-Stocked Pantry

When you're making desserts with minimal sugar and fat, good quality basic ingredients are a must. With virtually no butter and little sugar, the real flavor of everything else you put in a dessert really shines through. You won't find recipes in this book that will send you to specialty markets or online shopping, but do be sure to buy the best and freshest basic ingredients for making desserts.

Expand Your Stash of Sweeteners

Molasses, real maple syrup, honey, and brown sugar (the "brown" comes from molasses, which adds great earthy flavor) add more than just sweetness to recipes. Each one has its own unique flavor, and with molasses, maple syrup, and honey, the tastes can be infinitely different depending on the producer.

Use these flavor-boosters in recipes as well as for brushing on the tops of warm muffins, loaf breads, or cakes. If you taste a little sweetness on the top of baked goods, you can do with less sugar in the treat itself.

Another sweetener with loads of flavor is lower- or no-sugar preserves. These are made with half or none of the sugar of regular preserves, and they have brighter, fresher fruit flavor. A little of them goes a long way, too. Spoon them into the center of muffin batter before baking, smear onto toasted slices of loaf breads, or use instead of icing to spread between cake layers.

Or try another trick for topping desserts: use ordinary confectioners' sugar. A tiny bit—about 1 teaspoon—works like magic fairy dust, topping an entire cake, a batch of muffins, or a loaf bread with a sweet sprinkle of flavor.

The recipes in this book are designed to have enough sugar to provide the functional purposes of sugar (browning, tenderness, and volume), yet be low enough in carbs that they're easy to enjoy even when you are eating for good health. To artificially sweeten with success, I like to use Splenda® granular no-calorie sweetener. It functions best of all the artificial sweeteners when heated, and seems to have the least bitter aftertaste of other options on the market.

Fall in Love with Fruit

Because fruits contain natural sugars, they're already sweet, so in most instances you can use less sugar in a dessert made with fruit. Buy fruits that are in season and use them at their peak of ripeness. Berries, cherries, grapes, pineapples, and citrus fruits won't ripen after picking, so if these don't look good in the market, they're not going to improve with age. But, fruits like pears, figs, apricots, peaches, plums, and mangos will ripen in a few days on the counter. Any dessert will taste better made with perfectly ripe fruit.

Because frostings are high in fat, sugars, and calories, they should be a rare treat. But don't feel deprived. Use fruits as fresh, invigorating accompaniments to desserts instead of overly sweet frostings. One of many examples of how this works in these recipes is the Orange Polenta Cake on page 26. It's a deliciously simple cake on its own, but served with fresh orange segments in winter or fresh berries in summer, it is sublime. Use this trick with your own recipes to boost flavor and cut sugar, calories, and fat.

Make the Most of Nuts and Chocolate

Nuts and chocolate are a real treat when you're watching your fat and calorie intake, so make the best of the small amounts you do enjoy. Buy nuts that are not chopped for optimum freshness and flavor and store them in the freezer to extend their shelf life. Toasting them in the oven at 350°F for 5 to 8 minutes brings out their nuttiest flavors.

As much as everyone loves chocolate, it contains saturated fat. Even unsweetened dry cocoa has almost half a gram of saturated fat in a tablespoon. So, make the best of the little bit you use. Grating chocolate is an easy way to make a modest amount to go a long way. Topping cakes and puddings with a light sprinkle of grated semisweet or bittersweet chocolate delivers the flavor you crave with minimum fat and calories.

If you haven't discovered miniature chocolate chips, give them a try for muffins, loaf breads, and cookies. A small amount can fleck a dessert with great chocolate flavor. For a delicious drizzle on a cake, pie, or batch of muffins using a minimum of chocolate, chop about 1/2 an ounce of semisweet or bittersweet chocolate, place it in a resealable plastic bag, and drop the bag into a pot of hot water for a couple of minutes. Snip a tiny corner off the bag and drizzle on the melted chocolate.

Use Low Fat, Not No Fat

Fat-free cream cheese and sour cream tend to have a chalky texture and an artificial aftertaste. The reduced-fat versions certainly have more calories and fat, but a smaller serving will be more flavorful and satisfying than a dessert made with the fat-free versions.

Eliminate Trans Fat

Never use stick margarine or solid shortenings containing trans fat. Trans fat raises blood cholesterol and reduces the amount of good-for-your-heart LDLs. When a hard fat is used in the recipes in this book, it is trans-fat-free 67% vegetable oil butter-flavored spread. Look for the Smart Balance® brand—it works quite well in making flaky pie crusts and crispy cookies.

Make More Than Meringue

Meringue powder—also known as dried egg whites—is useful for making meringue toppings for pies, but also for lightening the texture of custards and pie fillings and for creating a light and delicious option to whipped cream (see page 82). You'll find it in the baking section of large supermarkets, in baking supply stores, or in discount stores that stock baking supplies.

Spice Things Up

Spices add wonderful flavors and aromas to desserts—but not if they've been in your pantry for years. Go through your spices and toss anything that's been around for more than a year. Replace them with the smallest possible sizes—buying the smaller size will help you keep a rotation of fresh spices in your pantry. And pay for the national brand spices—don't buy the discount brands. There really is a difference in taste.

Tools for Better Baking

A well-equipped kitchen makes making desserts—or anything else—a pleasure instead of a pain. Even if you make desserts infrequently, spending the time and money to stock up on quality basic equipment will help make the task easy and the sweets you bake look and taste great. Buy a few things at a time as your budget allows and soon enough, you'll have a kitchen well stocked for baking.

Proper Pans

Use shiny-surfaced, heavy-gauge aluminum baking pans. Aluminum conducts heat well and heats evenly for uniform browning. Pans with dark surfaces, including nonstick pans, tend to cause over-baking and excessive browning.

If they're not already part of your kitchen inventory, some smaller baking pans are a good investment. Because baked goods don't rise as much when you use less sugar, smaller pans make them seem more proportionate. A 9-inch loaf cake that's only 2 inches tall seems out of proportion, but bake the same batter in an 8-inch pan and your cake's relatively taller. You'll find enough uses for a couple of 8-inch round cake pans and an 8-inch loaf pan to make them well worth the expense.

Parchment Paper

Available in the baking section of most large supermarkets, parchment paper is indispensable for baking cakes and cookies. Taking the extra minute to line a pan with parchment paper will ensure that your cake comes out looking bakery-perfect. It's worth keeping parchment on hand to use for baking cookies to save on cleanup alone. Let the pan cool between batches, wipe off the parchment with paper towels, and use it again to bake the next batch of cookies—no pan washing required!

Pastry Brushes

Keep a few pastry brushes on hand to brush honey, molasses, or maple syrup onto warm baked goods. You will use a lot less of the high-carb, yet great-tasting sweets than you would by drizzling, and you'll get more even coverage. They're also indispensable for brushing flavorings onto ladyfingers or cakes and for making trifles or layered desserts.

Microplane® Grater

Lemon, orange, and lime zest add an unbelievable punch of flavor to endless types of desserts (not to mention savory foods, too). If you don't have one, invest about $12 in a Microplane® grater. These small graters were originally manufactured for use by woodworkers to shave away tiny slivers of wood. With a Microplane®, you can grate a tablespoon of beautiful thin strips of citrus zest in less than a minute. Use it for grating whole nutmeg and chocolate, too.

Offset Spatulas

A small offset spatula allows you to spread a thin, even layer of a frosting or a glaze onto cakes, and a larger one makes it easy to spread thick batters to an even thickness into a baking pan. You'll find lots of uses for these in your savory cooking, too, so it's worth having a couple on hand.

Cookie Scoop

If you bake a lot of cookies, a scoop will make the job quicker and easier. Finding one that's small enough for suitable portion control is not easy—most of the ones typically found in baking supply shops make saucer-sized cookies. Look for a two-teaspoon stainless steel scoop (called a #100 size).

Tips and Techniques for Perfection Every Time

Creating low-sugar, low-fat desserts is not that much different than making regular desserts, but there are a few pointers to keep in mind before you head for the kitchen.

Testing for Doneness

You can't count on the same timing and visual cues with low-sugar baking as with traditional baking. With less sugar, baking times are shorter, and because there is not as much browning, you can't always depend on the brownness of a cake or muffin to tell when it's done. Check baked goods 5 minutes before the indicated bake time in the recipe and insert a wooden toothpick into the center; when it comes out clean, with no clinging batter, the cake, loaf bread, or muffin is done. Try not to over-bake in order to retain as much moisture as possible.

A Perfect Pie Crust

The flavor and flakiness of the basic pastry crust used in pies and tarts in this book is excellent, but because it's made with less fat, you'll find it more delicate to work with than a crust made with an abundance of shortening or butter. Here's the simple secret to working with a low-fat crust: when rolling it out, place it between 2 sheets of waxed paper and rotate the paper often as you roll to create an even circle. Peel off the top piece of paper, invert the crust into the pie plate, and then gently peel away the top piece of wax paper.

Storing Baked Goods

Baked goods made with sugar substitutes lose moisture faster than those made with regular sugar, so they stale faster. A cake that might last a week made with sugar will only last a couple of days when made with a blend of sugar and granular no-calorie sweetener.

Plan on freezing extra muffins and quick breads that you don't intend to serve right away. Freezing will slow moisture loss better than room temperature storage. Also, muffins and cupcakes will stay fresh longer if they are baked in paper muffin liners coated with cooking spray. The paper liner helps keep the moisture in and protects them against staling.

THE DESSERTS IN THIS BOOK were created to be a part of moments that make your life special. Whether it's a weekend brunch with family, a quick breakfast muffin with your spouse, or a birthday celebration for a friend, you'll find delicious treats here to share with friends and family that they will enjoy just as much as you do.

Great Cakes

Lemon–Spice Carrot Cake with Cream Cheese Frosting

Makes 24 servings • Serving size: 1 (3 × 1 1/2-inch) piece

Fresh lemon gives this classic sheet cake, shown on the front cover,
a flavorful lift. It's easy to make, too—no mixer required.

Lemon-Spice Carrot Cake

1 1/2 cups all-purpose flour

1 1/2 cups whole wheat flour

3/4 cup granulated sugar

3/4 cup granular no-calorie sweetener

2 teaspoons baking powder

1 teaspoon baking soda

1 teaspoon ground cinnamon

1 teaspoon ground ginger

1/2 teaspoon ground nutmeg

1/4 teaspoon salt

2 (6-ounce) containers plain fat-free yogurt

1/4 cup canola oil

2 large eggs

1 tablespoon fresh grated lemon zest

2 cups finely shredded carrots
(about 4 medium carrots)

Cream Cheese Frosting

1 cup granulated sugar

1 cup granular no-calorie sweetener

2/3 cup all-purpose flour

1 cup fat-free milk

6 ounces reduced-fat cream cheese,
cut into cubes

3 tablespoons fresh lemon juice

Garnish

Thin strips lemon peel (optional)

Make Cake

1. Preheat the oven to 350°F. Coat a 13 × 9-inch baking pan with cooking spray and set aside.

2. Combine the all-purpose flour, whole wheat flour, sugar, no-calorie sweetener, baking powder, baking soda, cinnamon, ginger, nutmeg, and salt in a large bowl and whisk to mix well. Set aside.

3. Combine the yogurt, oil, eggs, and lemon zest in a medium bowl and whisk until smooth. Add the oil mixture to the flour mixture and stir just until moistened. Stir in the carrots. (Batter will be very thick.)

4. Spoon the batter into the prepared pan and smooth the top. Bake 25 to 30 minutes or until a wooden toothpick inserted in the center of the cake comes out clean.

5. Cool the cake in the pan on a wire rack for 10 minutes. Remove from the pan and cool completely on the wire rack.

Make Frosting

1. Combine the sugar, no-calorie sweetener, flour, and milk in a saucepan and whisk until smooth. Cook over medium-high heat, whisking constantly, for 5 minutes until the mixture comes to a boil and becomes extremely thick.

2. Remove from the heat and add the cream cheese, stirring until the cream cheese melts. Spoon the frosting into a medium bowl and cover the surface with plastic wrap. Cool to room temperature and stir in the lemon juice.

3. Spread the frosting over the top of the cake. Garnish each serving with thin strips of lemon peel, if desired. The cake can be covered in an airtight container and stored in the refrigerator up to 3 days.

Exchanges: 2 Carbohydrate • 1/2 Fat
Calories 165, Calories from Fat 40, Total Fat 5 g, Saturated Fat 1 g, Cholesterol 25 mg, Sodium 165 mg, Total Carbohydrate 27 g, Dietary Fiber 2 g, Sugars 12 g, Protein 5 g.

CHOCOLATE-DRIZZLED PEANUT BUTTER CAKE

Makes 9 servings • Serving size: 1 (2 1/2-inch) square

For a lunch box, an after school treat, a bake sale, or a coffee break, this cake is a pleasing sweet for peanut butter lovers of all ages.

1 cup all-purpose flour

1 teaspoon baking powder

1/2 teaspoon baking soda

1/8 teaspoon salt

1/4 cup natural peanut butter

3 tablespoons canola oil

1/3 cup granular no-calorie sweetener

1/3 cup light brown sugar

1 large egg

3/4 cup low-fat buttermilk

1 teaspoon vanilla extract

1/2 ounce semisweet chocolate baking bar, chopped

1. Preheat the oven to 350°F. Coat an 8 × 8-inch baking pan with cooking spray and set aside.
2. Combine the flour, baking powder, baking soda, and salt in a medium bowl and whisk to mix well. Set aside.
3. Combine the peanut butter and oil in a medium bowl and beat at medium speed until smooth. Beat in the no-calorie sweetener and brown sugar. Beat in the egg. Add the flour mixture and buttermilk alternately to the peanut butter mixture, beginning and ending with the flour mixture, beating well after each addition. Beat in the vanilla.
4. Spoon the batter into the prepared pan and smooth the top. Bake 20 to 25 minutes or until a wooden toothpick inserted in the center of the cake comes out clean. Cool the cake in the pan on a wire rack for 10 minutes. Remove from the pan and cool completely on the rack.
5. Place the chocolate in a small resealable zip-top bag and seal. Place the bag in a saucepan of hot water. Let stand 5 minutes or until the chocolate melts. Snip a tiny corner from bag and drizzle chocolate over the cake. The cake can be covered in an airtight container and stored at room temperature up to 3 days.

Exchanges: 1 1/2 Carbohydrate • 2 Fat
Calories 193, Calories from Fat 86, Total Fat 10 g, Saturated Fat 1 g, Cholesterol 24 mg, Sodium 204 mg, Total Carbohydrate 23 g, Dietary Fiber 1 g, Sugars 11 g, Protein 5 g.

Blueberry–Lemon Buttermilk Cake

Makes 8 servings • Serving size: 1 slice

Wonderfully moist and so easy to make, this yummy cake makes a nice
dessert choice for brunch, tea, or a weeknight supper.

1 1/2 cups all-purpose flour

1 teaspoon baking powder

1/2 teaspoon baking soda

1/4 teaspoon salt

3/4 cup low-fat buttermilk

1/2 cup granulated sugar

1/4 cup granular
no-calorie sweetener

1/4 cup canola oil

1 large egg

1 tablespoon fresh grated
lemon zest

1 cup fresh blueberries, or
frozen unthawed blueberries

1 teaspoon
confectioners' sugar

1. Preheat the oven to 350°F. Line an 8-inch round cake pan with parchment paper and coat the paper and sides of the pan with cooking spray. Set aside.

2. Combine the flour, baking powder, baking soda, and salt in a medium bowl and whisk to mix well. Set aside.

3. Combine the buttermilk, sugar, no-calorie sweetener, oil, egg, and lemon zest in a medium bowl and whisk until smooth. Add the buttermilk mixture to the flour mixture, whisking until a smooth batter forms. Gently stir in the blueberries.

4. Spoon the batter into the prepared pan. Bake 25 to 30 minutes or until a wooden toothpick inserted in the center of the cake comes out clean. Cool the cake in the pan on a wire rack for 10 minutes. Run a knife around the edge of the cake, remove from the pan, discarding parchment paper, and cool completely on the wire rack. Just before serving, place confectioners' sugar in a small fine-mesh sieve and sprinkle over the cake. The cake is best on the day it is made.

Exchanges: 2 1/2 Carbohydrate • 1 Fat
Calories 230, Calories from Fat 70, Total Fat 8 g, Saturated Fat 1 g, Cholesterol 25 mg, Sodium 230 mg, Total Carbohydrate 35 g, Dietary Fiber 1 g, Sugars 17 g, Protein 4 g.

Mocha Fudge Sheet Cake

Makes 24 servings • Serving size: 1 (3 × 1 1/2-inch) piece

For a bake sale, a casual supper, or a family reunion, nothing beats a great chocolate cake. The frosting goes on while it's warm, so make it while the cake bakes and you'll have a welcome treat that's complete in less than an hour.

Mocha Fudge Cake

3 cups all-purpose flour

1 cup granulated sugar

3/4 cup granular no-calorie sweetener

1 cup unsweetened cocoa

2 teaspoons baking powder

2 teaspoons baking soda

1/4 teaspoon salt

2 cups strong brewed coffee, cooled

1/2 cup canola oil

2 teaspoons vanilla extract

Chocolate Frosting

1/2 cup granulated sugar

1/2 cup granular no-calorie sweetener

1/3 cup all-purpose flour

3/4 cup fat-free milk

2 (1-ounce) squares unsweetened chocolate, chopped

1 1/2 teaspoons vanilla extract

Make Cake

1. Preheat the oven to 325°F. Coat a 13 × 9-inch baking pan with cooking spray and set aside.

2. Combine the flour, sugar, no-calorie sweetener, cocoa, baking powder, baking soda, and salt in a large bowl and whisk to mix well. Set aside.

3. Combine the coffee, oil, and vanilla in a medium bowl. Add the coffee mixture to the flour mixture and stir just until moistened.

4. Spoon the batter into the prepared pan and smooth the top. Bake for 25 to 28 minutes or until a wooden toothpick inserted in the center of the cake comes out clean. Cool in a pan on a wire rack for 20 minutes.

5. Spread Chocolate Frosting over the warm cake. Cool completely in the pan on the wire rack. The cake can be covered in an airtight container and stored in the refrigerator up to 3 days.

Make Frosting

1. Combine the sugar, no-calorie sweetener, flour, and milk in a saucepan and whisk until smooth. Cook over medium-high heat, whisking constantly, for 5 minutes until the mixture comes to a boil and thickens to pudding consistency.

2. Remove from the heat and add the chocolate, stirring until the chocolate melts. Spoon the frosting into a medium bowl and let stand 10 to 15 minutes to cool and thicken slightly. Stir in the vanilla and spoon onto the cake while warm.

Variation

To use the cake recipe to make Mocha Fudge Cupcakes, line 30 muffin cups with paper liners and coat the liners with cooking spray. Spoon the batter into prepared cups and bake at 350°F for 12 to 15 minutes or until a wooden toothpick inserted into one of the cupcakes comes out clean. Spread Chocolate Frosting evenly over warm cupcakes.

Exchanges: 2 Carbohydrate • 1 Fat
Calories 182, Calories from Fat 58, Total Fat 6 g, Saturated Fat 1 g, Cholesterol 0 mg, Sodium 166 mg, Total Carbohydrate 30 g, Dietary Fiber 2 g, Sugars 15 g, Protein 3 g.

Havana Banana Cake

Makes 8 servings • Serving size: 1 slice

This update on upside-down cake makes a striking presentation with the caramelized bananas on top of the cake. A splash of rum adds a taste of the tropics.

2 tablespoons 67% vegetable oil butter-flavored spread, melted

2 tablespoons light brown sugar

1 medium ripe banana, thinly sliced on the diagonal

1 cup all-purpose flour

1/2 cup granulated sugar

1 teaspoon baking powder

1/2 teaspoon baking soda

1/2 teaspoon ground cinnamon

1/4 teaspoon salt

1/2 cup mashed ripe banana (about 1 medium banana)

1/2 cup low-fat buttermilk

2 tablespoons canola oil

2 tablespoons dark rum or 1 teaspoon rum extract

1 large egg

1. Preheat the oven to 350°F.

2. Coat the sides of an 8-inch round cake pan with cooking spray. Pour the butter-flavored spread into the pan, tilting to coat the bottom. Sprinkle the brown sugar evenly in the pan and arrange the banana slices in a single layer over the sugar.

3. Combine the flour, granulated sugar, baking powder, baking soda, cinnamon, and salt in a large bowl and whisk to mix well. Set aside. Combine the mashed banana, buttermilk, oil, rum, and egg in a medium bowl and whisk until the mixture is smooth. Add the banana mixture to the flour mixture and stir until moistened.

4. Spoon the batter over the sliced bananas. Bake 30 to 35 minutes or until a wooden toothpick inserted in the center of the cake comes out clean. Immediately invert the cake onto a serving plate. Let cool 10 minutes before slicing. Serve warm or at room temperature. The cake is best on the day it is made.

Exchanges: 2 1/2 Carbohydrate • 1 Fat
Calories 214, Calories from Fat 62, Total Fat 7 g, Saturated Fat 1 g, Cholesterol 27 mg, Sodium 246 mg, Total Carbohydrate 36 g, Dietary Fiber 1 g, Sugars 20 g, Protein 3 g.

CRANBERRY BRUNCH CAKE

Makes 8 servings • Serving size: 1 slice

This moist, berry-studded cake gets extra flavor and tenderness from a
generous portion of yogurt. Serve it at brunch or to finish a casual winter meal.
If you use frozen cranberries, you don't have to thaw them first.

1 1/2 cups cake flour

1 1/2 teaspoons baking powder

1/2 teaspoon baking soda

1/4 teaspoon salt

1/3 cup granulated sugar

1/3 cup granular no-calorie sweetener

2 tablespoons 67% vegetable oil butter-flavored spread, at room temperature

1 large egg

1 cup plain fat-free yogurt

1 teaspoon vanilla extract

1 cup fresh cranberries or frozen cranberries, unthawed

1 teaspoon confectioners' sugar

1. Preheat the oven to 350°F. Coat an 8-inch round cake pan with cooking spray. Set aside.

2. Combine the flour, baking powder, baking soda, and salt in a medium bowl and whisk to mix well. Set aside.

3. Combine the sugar, no-calorie sweetener, and butter-flavored spread in a large bowl and beat at medium speed until mixture resembles coarse cornmeal. Beat in the egg.

4. Add the flour mixture to the sugar mixture, alternating with the yogurt, beginning and ending with the flour mixture. Beat in the vanilla. Gently stir in the cranberries.

5. Spoon the batter into the prepared pan. Bake 25 to 30 minutes or until a wooden toothpick inserted in the center of the cake comes out clean.

6. Cool in the pan on a rack for 10 minutes. Remove from the pan and cool completely on the wire rack. Just before serving, place the confectioners' sugar in a small fine-mesh sieve and sprinkle over the cake. The cake is best on the day it is made.

Exchanges: 2 Carbohydrate • 1/2 Fat
Calories 183, Calories from Fat 29, Total Fat 3 g, Saturated Fat 1 g, Cholesterol 29 mg, Sodium 272 mg, Total Carbohydrate 34 g, Dietary Fiber 1 g, Sugars 13 g, Protein 4 g.

RASPBERRY–YOGURT CAKE

Makes 8 servings • Serving size: 1 slice

Yogurt gives this simple cake a wonderful tang and tenderness.
Fresh raspberries make it irresistible. Try it with blueberries, too.

1 cup all-purpose flour

1 teaspoon baking powder

1/2 teaspoon baking soda

1/4 teaspoon salt

1/2 cup granulated sugar

3/4 cup plain fat-free yogurt

2 tablespoons canola oil

1 large egg

2 teaspoons vanilla extract

1 cup fresh raspberries, or
frozen unthawed raspberries

1. Preheat the oven to 350°F. Coat an 8-inch round cake pan with cooking spray and set aside.

2. Combine the flour, baking powder, baking soda, and salt in a medium bowl and whisk to mix well. Set aside.

3. Combine the sugar, yogurt, oil, egg, and vanilla in a medium bowl and whisk until smooth. Add the sugar mixture to the flour mixture, stirring just until a moist batter forms.

4. Spoon the batter into the prepared pan and sprinkle the top evenly with raspberries. Bake 30 to 35 minutes or until the cake is lightly browned and the top springs back when lightly touched in the center. Cool the cake in the pan on a wire rack for 10 minutes before slicing. Serve the cake from the pan, warm or at room temperature. The cake is best on the day it is made.

Exchanges: 2 Carbohydrate • 1/2 Fat
Calories 167, Calories from Fat 40, Total Fat 4 g, Saturated Fat 1 g, Cholesterol 28 mg, Sodium 221 mg, Total Carbohydrate 28 g, Dietary Fiber 1 g, Sugars 15 g, Protein 4 g.

Old-Fashioned Apple Spice Cake

Makes 8 servings • Serving size: 1 slice

Cooking the apples allows their sugars to caramelize, adding more flavor and softening them to yield a moist-textured cake. Ripe Bartlett pears make a fine substitute for the apples.

1 tablespoon plus 1/4 cup canola oil, divided use

2 large Golden Delicious apples, peeled and chopped

1 cup all-purpose flour

1 cup whole wheat flour

1 teaspoon baking powder

2 teaspoons ground cinnamon

1/2 teaspoon baking soda

1/4 teaspoon salt

1/4 teaspoon ground cloves

1 cup plain low-fat yogurt

1/2 cup granulated sugar

1/4 cup granular no-calorie sweetener

1 large egg

2 teaspoons vanilla extract

1. Preheat the oven to 350°F. Coat an 8-inch round cake pan with cooking spray. Set aside.

2. Heat 1 tablespoon of the oil in a large nonstick skillet over medium-high heat. Add the apples and cook 5 minutes, stirring often, until softened and lightly browned. Set aside.

3. Combine the all-purpose flour, whole wheat flour, baking powder, cinnamon, baking soda, salt, and cloves in a large bowl and whisk to mix well. Combine the yogurt, sugar, no-calorie sweetener, remaining 1/4 cup oil, egg, and vanilla in a medium bowl and whisk to mix well. Add the yogurt mixture and the apples to the flour mixture and stir until well combined. (Batter will be very thick.)

4. Spoon the batter into the prepared pan, smooth the top, and bake 35 to 40 minutes, until the edge is lightly browned and a wooden toothpick inserted in the center comes out clean. Cool the cake in the pan on a wire rack for 10 minutes. Remove from the pan and cool completely on the wire rack. The cake is best on the day it is made.

Exchanges: 3 Carbohydrate • 1 1/2 Fat
Calories 293, Calories from Fat 94, Total Fat 10 g, Saturated Fat 1 g, Cholesterol 28 mg, Sodium 227 mg, Total Carbohydrate 45 g, Dietary Fiber 3 g, Sugars 21 g, Protein 6 g.

ALMOND CAKE WITH ROASTED PEACHES

Makes 12 servings • Serving size: 1 slice cake and 1/4 peach

It's essential to have the eggs and milk at room temperature before making this cake to prevent the almond paste from forming lumps in the batter.

Almond Cake

1 1/2 cups all-purpose flour

1 1/2 teaspoons baking powder

1/4 teaspoon salt

1/2 cup granulated sugar

1/3 cup granular no-calorie sweetener

1/3 cup canola oil

7 ounces almond paste, cut into small pieces

2 large eggs, at room temperature

1/4 cup 1% low-fat milk, at room temperature

2 teaspoons vanilla extract

Roasted Peaches

3 medium peaches, peeled, pitted, and quartered

1 tablespoon canola oil

Make Cake

1. Preheat the oven to 350°F. Line the bottom of a 9-inch round cake pan with parchment paper and coat the paper and sides of the pan with cooking spray. Set aside.

2. Combine the flour, baking powder, and salt in a medium bowl and whisk to mix well. Set aside.

3. Combine the sugar, no-calorie sweetener, and oil in a large bowl and beat at medium speed until well combined. Beat in the almond paste, a few pieces at a time, beating well after each addition, until mixture is smooth. Beat in the eggs, one at a time. Add the milk and beat until smooth. Beat in the vanilla. Add the flour mixture and beat at low speed just until a smooth batter forms.

4. Spoon the batter into the prepared pan and smooth the top. Bake 25 to 30 minutes or until a wooden toothpick inserted in the center of the cake comes out clean. Cool the cake in the pan on a wire rack for 5 minutes. Run a knife around the edge of the cake, remove the cake from the pan, discarding parchment paper, and cool completely on the wire rack.

Make Peaches

1. Preheat the oven to 400°F. Combine the peaches and oil in a large bowl and toss to coat. Place the peaches in a single layer in a large baking pan.

2. Bake, stirring once, 15 to 20 minutes or until peaches are lightly browned and softened.

3. Serve the cake with Roasted Peaches. The cake can be covered in an airtight container and stored at room temperature up to 1 day.

Exchanges: 2 Carbohydrate • 2 1/2 Fat
Calories 262, Calories from Fat 116, Total Fat 13 g, Saturated Fat 1 g, Cholesterol 36 mg, Sodium 110 mg, Total Carbohydrate 33 g, Dietary Fiber 2 g, Sugars 19 g, Protein 5 g.

Orange–Polenta Cake

Makes 10 servings • Serving size: 1 slice with 1/4 cup orange segments

This sophisticated dessert begs for fresh fruit to balance the richness of the cake. In fall and winter, serve it with orange segments. When fresh berries are in season, use those instead.

1 cup yellow cornmeal (not cornmeal mix)

3/4 cup all-purpose flour

1/2 cup granulated sugar

1/2 cup granular no-calorie sweetener

2/3 cup low-fat buttermilk

1/3 cup extra-virgin olive oil

1/2 teaspoon baking soda

1/4 teaspoon salt

2 large eggs

2 teaspoons vanilla extract

1 tablespoon fresh grated orange zest

4 large navel or Valencia oranges

1. Preheat the oven to 350°F. Line the bottom of an 8-inch round cake pan with parchment paper. Coat the paper and sides of the pan with cooking spray. Set aside.

2. Combine the cornmeal, flour, sugar, no-calorie sweetener, buttermilk, oil, baking soda, salt, and eggs in a large bowl and beat at medium speed for 2 to 3 minutes or until the batter is smooth. Beat in the vanilla and stir in the orange zest. Pour the batter into the prepared pan and bake 25 to 30 minutes, or until a wooden toothpick inserted in the center comes out clean.

3. While the cake bakes, prepare the orange segments. Cut a thin slice from the top and bottom of each of the oranges, exposing the flesh. Stand each orange upright, and using a sharp knife, thickly cut off the peel, following the contour of the fruit and removing all the white pith and membrane. Holding the orange over a medium bowl, carefully cut along both sides of each section to free it from the membrane. Discard any seeds and let the sections fall into the bowl.

4. Cool the cake in the pan on a wire rack for 10 minutes. Remove from the pan, discard the parchment, and cool completely on the wire rack. Serve the cake with the orange segments. The cake can be covered in an airtight container and stored at room temperature up to 1 day.

Exchanges: 2 1/2 Carbohydrate • 1 1/2 Fat
Calories 250, Calories from Fat 78, Total Fat 9 g, Saturated Fat 1 g, Cholesterol 43 mg, Sodium 153 mg, Total Carbohydrate 39 g, Dietary Fiber 3 g, Sugars 19 g, Protein 5 g.

Walnut Spice Cake with Maple Sauce

Makes 12 servings • Serving size: 1 slice cake with 2 tablespoons sauce

Finely ground walnuts enrich this cake with nutty flavor.
Serve the maple sauce with other cakes, or drizzle it over fresh fruit.

Walnut Spice Cake

1/3 cup chopped walnuts

1/2 cup granulated sugar

1/2 cup granular no-calorie sweetener

2 cups all-purpose flour

2 teaspoons baking powder

1/2 teaspoon baking soda

1 teaspoon ground ginger

1 teaspoon ground cinnamon

1/2 teaspoon ground cloves

1/4 teaspoon salt

1/4 cup 67% vegetable oil butter-flavored spread, at room temperature

1/4 cup maple syrup

1 large egg

1 cup low-fat buttermilk

2 teaspoons vanilla extract

Maple Sauce

1 (12-ounce) can fat-free evaporated milk

3 tablespoons all-purpose flour

2 tablespoons granular no-calorie sweetener

3 tablespoons maple syrup

Make Cake

1. Preheat the oven to 350°F. Place the walnuts in a small baking pan and bake, stirring once, 5 to 8 minutes or until lightly toasted. Set aside to cool. Maintain the oven temperature.

2. Line the bottom of a 9-inch round cake pan with parchment paper. Coat the paper and sides of the pan with cooking spray and set aside.

3. Combine the walnuts, sugar, and no-calorie sweetener in a food processor and process until the nuts are finely ground. Set aside.

4. Combine the flour, baking powder, baking soda, ginger, cinnamon, cloves, and salt in a medium bowl and whisk to mix well. Set aside.

5. Combine the butter-flavored spread and maple syrup in a large bowl and beat at medium speed until the mixture is smooth. Beat in the egg. Add the flour mixture and buttermilk alternately to the butter-flavored spread mixture, beginning and ending with the flour mixture, beating well after each addition. Beat in the vanilla. Add the walnut mixture and beat at low speed just until blended.

6. Spoon the batter into the prepared pan. Bake 30 to 35 minutes or until a wooden toothpick inserted in center of cake comes out clean. Cool the cake in the pan on a wire rack for 10 minutes. Remove from the pan, discard the parchment, and cool completely on the wire rack. Serve with the Maple Sauce. The cake can be covered in an airtight container and stored at room temperature up to 2 days.

Make Sauce

1. Combine the evaporated milk, flour, and no-calorie sweetener in a medium saucepan and whisk until the mixture is smooth. Cook over medium heat, 4 to 5 minutes, stirring constantly, until the mixture comes to a boil and thickens.

2. Transfer to a medium bowl and cover the surface of the sauce with plastic wrap to prevent a skin from forming. Cool to room temperature and stir in the maple syrup. The sauce can be stored in the refrigerator up to 3 days.

Exchanges: 2 1/2 Carbohydrate • 1 Fat
Calories 243, Calories from Fat 56, Total Fat 6 g, Saturated Fat 1 g, Cholesterol 20 mg, Sodium 258 mg, Total Carbohydrate 40 g, Dietary Fiber 1 g, Sugars 22 g, Protein 7 g.

Flourless Hazelnut–Orange Cake

Makes 8 servings • Serving size: 1 slice

Serve this simple yet sophisticated cake on its own or with fresh berries, orange segments, or the Maple–Cider Fruit Compote on page 151.

3/4 cup hazelnuts	1 tablespoon fresh grated orange zest
4 large eggs, separated	1/4 teaspoon cream of tartar
1/2 cup granulated sugar	1/2 teaspoon vanilla extract
1/2 cup granular no-calorie sweetener	1 teaspoon confectioners' sugar

1. Preheat the oven to 350°F.

2. Place the hazelnuts in a small bowl and cover with hot water. Let stand 1 minute, then drain. Place the hazelnuts in a small baking pan and bake 8 to 10 minutes, stirring once, until the skins begin to flake. Maintain the oven temperature.

3. Working with a few nuts at a time, place them in a kitchen towel and rub off the skins. Place the cooled hazelnuts in a food processor and process until finely ground. Set aside.

4. Line the bottom of an 8-inch round cake pan with parchment paper. Coat the paper and sides of the pan with cooking spray and set aside.

5. Combine the egg yolks, sugar, and no-calorie sweetener in a large bowl and beat at medium speed until fluffy and pale yellow in color. Stir in the hazelnuts and orange zest.

6. Place the egg whites and cream of tartar in a large bowl and beat at high speed until stiff peaks form. Fold the egg white mixture into the hazelnut mixture in four additions, mixing until no white streaks remain. Spoon the batter into the prepared pan and smooth the top. Bake 20 to 25 minutes or until the center of the cake is firm to the touch.

7. Cool the cake in the pan on a wire rack for 10 minutes. Remove from the pan, discard the parchment paper, and cool completely on the wire rack. Place the confectioners' sugar in a small fine-mesh sieve and sprinkle over the cake. The cake can be covered in an airtight container and stored at room temperature up to 1 day.

Exchanges: 1 Carbohydrate • 2 Fat
Calories 162, Calories from Fat 81, Total Fat 9 g, Saturated Fat 1 g, Cholesterol 106 mg, Sodium 35 mg, Total Carbohydrate 17 g, Dietary Fiber 1 g, Sugars 15 g, Protein 5 g.

Orange-Glazed Pumpkin Bundt Cake

Makes 10 servings • Serving size: 1 slice

When you tire of eating pumpkin pie in the autumn, try this lightly spiced, orange-glazed cake. It's nice and moist, so you can make it a day ahead if you need a jump start on getting ready for company.

1 cup all-purpose flour

1/2 cup whole wheat flour

2 teaspoons pumpkin pie spice

1 teaspoon baking powder

1/2 teaspoon baking soda

1/4 teaspoon salt

1/4 cup 67% vegetable oil butter-flavored spread, at room temperature

1/2 cup granular no-calorie sweetener

1/2 cup light brown sugar

1 cup solid-pack pumpkin (not pumpkin pie filling)

1 large egg

1/2 cup low-fat buttermilk

2 teaspoons vanilla extract

1/3 cup confectioners' sugar

2 to 3 teaspoons orange juice

1. Preheat the oven to 350°F. Coat a 6-cup Bundt pan with cooking spray and set aside.

2. Combine the all-purpose flour, whole wheat flour, pumpkin pie spice, baking powder, baking soda, and salt in a medium bowl and whisk to mix well. Set aside.

3. Combine the butter-flavored spread, no-calorie sweetener, and brown sugar in a large bowl and beat at medium speed until well mixed. Beat in the pumpkin and egg. Reduce speed to low and beat in the flour mixture. Beat in the buttermilk and vanilla, just until moistened.

4. Spoon the batter into the prepared pan. Bake 25 to 30 minutes or until a wooden toothpick inserted in the center of the cake comes out clean. Cool the cake in the pan on a wire rack for 10 minutes. Remove the cake from the pan and cool completely on the wire rack.

5. Combine the confectioners' sugar and 2 teaspoons of the orange juice in a small bowl, stirring until well mixed. Stir in additional orange juice, a few drops at a time, until the desired drizzling consistency is reached. Drizzle over the cooled cake. The cake can be covered in an airtight container and stored at room temperature up to 2 days.

Exchanges: 2 Carbohydrate • 1 Fat
Calories 186, Calories from Fat 42, Total Fat 5 g, Saturated Fat 1 g, Cholesterol 22 mg, Sodium 220 mg, Total Carbohydrate 33 g, Dietary Fiber 2 g, Sugars 17 g, Protein 3 g.

Date Spice Cake

Makes 16 servings • Serving size: 1 (1/2-inch) slice

When this cake is in the oven, the house is filled with the comforting aroma of spices.
It's a thoughtful holiday gift or a welcome treat on a brisk fall afternoon.

1 1/4 cups all-purpose flour

3/4 cup whole wheat flour

2 teaspoons baking powder

1 teaspoon baking soda

1 teaspoon ground cinnamon

1/2 teaspoon ground nutmeg

1/4 teaspoon ground cloves

1/4 teaspoon salt

1/3 cup 67% vegetable oil butter-flavored spread, at room temperature

1/2 cup granular no-calorie sweetener

1/2 cup light brown sugar

2 large eggs

1 cup low-fat buttermilk

1 teaspoon vanilla extract

3/4 cup pitted dates, chopped

1. Preheat the oven to 350°F. Coat an 8 × 4-inch loaf pan with cooking spray. Set aside.

2. Combine the all-purpose flour, whole wheat flour, baking powder, baking soda, cinnamon, nutmeg, cloves, and salt in a medium bowl and whisk to mix well. Set aside.

3. Combine the butter-flavored spread, no-calorie sweetener, and brown sugar in a large bowl and beat at medium speed until fluffy. Beat in the eggs one a time.

4. Add the flour mixture and buttermilk alternately to the butter-flavored spread mixture, beginning and ending with the flour mixture, beating well after each addition. Beat in the vanilla. Stir in the dates. Spoon the batter into the prepared pan and smooth the top. Bake 35 to 40 minutes or until a wooden toothpick inserted in the center of the cake comes out clean.

5. Cool in the pan on a wire rack for 10 minutes. Remove from the pan. Cool completely on the rack. The cake can be stored in an airtight container at room temperature for up to 3 days.

Exchanges: 2 Carbohydrate
Calories 152, Calories from Fat 37, Total Fat 4 g, Saturated Fat 1 g, Cholesterol 27 mg, Sodium 219 mg, Total Carbohydrate 26 g, Dietary Fiber 2 g, Sugars 14 g, Protein 3 g.

ORANGE–CARROT PICNIC CAKE

Makes 16 servings • Serving size: 1 slice

If you've got a shredding attachment on your food processor, this recipe is a snap. If not, think of shredding the carrots as an exercise in building upper body strength! It's a fantastically moist cake, flavored with fragrant spices and fresh orange zest—a definite keeper.

1 1/4 cups all-purpose flour

3/4 cup whole wheat flour

2 teaspoons baking powder

1 teaspoon baking soda

2 teaspoons ground cinnamon

1/4 teaspoon salt

3/4 cup granulated sugar

3/4 cup granular no-calorie sweetener

1/2 cup canola oil

1/2 cup reduced-fat mayonnaise

2 large eggs

3 cups finely shredded carrots (about 6 medium carrots)

1/2 cup chopped pecans

2 teaspoons fresh grated orange zest

1. Preheat the oven to 350°F. Coat a 10- or 12-cup Bundt pan with cooking spray and set aside.

2. Combine the all-purpose flour, whole wheat flour, baking powder, baking soda, cinnamon, and salt in a large bowl and whisk to mix well. Set aside.

3. Combine the sugar, no-calorie sweetener, oil, mayonnaise, and eggs in a medium bowl and whisk until smooth. Add the sugar mixture to the flour mixture and stir until the mixture is smooth. Stir in the carrots, pecans, and orange zest.

4. Spoon the batter into the prepared pan and smooth the top. Bake 35 to 40 minutes or until a wooden toothpick inserted in the center of the cake comes out clean. Cool in the pan on a wire rack for 10 minutes. Remove from the pan and cool completely on the wire rack. The cake can be stored in an airtight container at room temperature up to 2 days.

Exchanges: 2 Carbohydrate • 2 Fat

Calories 226, Calories from Fat 115, Total Fat 13 g, Saturated Fat 1 g, Cholesterol 29 mg, Sodium 254 mg, Total Carbohydrate 26 g, Dietary Fiber 2 g, Sugars 12 g, Protein 3 g.

GINGERY GINGERBREAD CAKE

Makes 16 servings • Serving size: 1 slice

Ginger ale, crystallized ginger, and ground ginger
give this cake a triple punch of flavor.

1 cup diet ginger ale, at room temperature

1/4 cup molasses

2 teaspoons baking soda

2 cups all-purpose flour

1/2 cup minced crystallized ginger

1 tablespoon ground ginger

2 teaspoons baking powder

1 teaspoon ground cinnamon

1/4 teaspoon ground nutmeg

1/4 teaspoon ground cloves

1/4 teaspoon salt

1/2 cup granular no-calorie sweetener

1/4 cup granulated sugar

1/4 cup light brown sugar

1/2 cup canola oil

2 large eggs

1/4 cup confectioners' sugar

2 to 3 teaspoons fresh lemon juice

1. Preheat the oven to 350°F. Coat a 10- or 12-cup Bundt pan with cooking spray and set aside.

2. Combine the ginger ale, molasses, and baking soda in a medium bowl and stir to mix well. Set aside. Combine the flour, crystallized ginger, ground ginger, baking powder, cinnamon, nutmeg, cloves, and salt in a large bowl and whisk to mix well. Set aside.

3. Combine the no-calorie sweetener, granulated sugar, brown sugar, oil, and eggs in a medium bowl and whisk to mix well. Slowly whisk the ginger ale mixture into the no-calorie sweetener mixture. Add the ginger ale mixture to the flour mixture, stirring until a smooth batter forms.

4. Spoon the batter into the prepared pan. Bake 30 to 35 minutes or until a wooden toothpick inserted in the center of the cake comes out clean. Cool the cake in the pan on a wire rack for 10 minutes. Remove the cake from the pan and cool completely on the wire rack.

5. Combine the confectioners' sugar and 2 teaspoons of the lemon juice in a small bowl, stirring until well mixed. Stir in additional lemon juice, a few drops at a time, until the desired drizzling consistency is reached. Drizzle the mixture over the cooled cake. The cake can be covered in an airtight container and stored at room temperature up to 2 days.

Exchanges: 2 Carbohydrate • 1 Fat
Calories 195, Calories from Fat 69, Total Fat 8 g, Saturated Fat 1 g, Cholesterol 26 mg, Sodium 254 mg, Total Carbohydrate 30 g, Dietary Fiber 1 g, Sugars 16 g, Protein 2 g.

CHARMING CHOCOLATE BUNDT CAKE

Makes 10 servings • Serving size: 1 slice

Baked in a small Bundt pan and drizzled with glossy chocolate syrup,
this cake is almost too cute to eat. Almost.

1 cup all-purpose flour

1/2 cup unsweetened cocoa

1 teaspoon baking powder

1/2 teaspoon baking soda

1/4 teaspoon salt

1/4 cup canola oil

3 large eggs

1/2 cup granulated sugar

1/2 cup granular no-calorie sweetener

1/2 cup low-fat buttermilk

1 teaspoon vanilla extract

2 tablespoons sugar-free chocolate syrup

1. Preheat the oven to 350°F. Coat a 6-cup Bundt pan with cooking spray. Set aside.

2. Combine the flour, cocoa, baking powder, baking soda, and salt in a medium bowl and whisk to mix well. Set aside.

3. Combine the oil and eggs in a large bowl and beat at medium speed until well mixed. Gradually beat in the sugar and no-calorie sweetener. Add the flour mixture and beat at low speed until smooth. Beat in the buttermilk and vanilla.

4. Spoon the batter into the prepared pan. Bake 25 to 30 minutes or until a wooden toothpick inserted in the center of the cake comes out clean. Cool the cake in the pan on a wire rack for 10 minutes. Remove the cake from the pan and drizzle the warm cake with syrup. Serve warm or at room temperature. The cake can be stored in an airtight container at room temperature up to 2 days.

Exchanges: 2 Carbohydrate • 1 Fat
Calories 185, Calories from Fat 70, Total Fat 8 g, Saturated Fat 1 g, Cholesterol 64 mg, Sodium 195 mg, Total Carbohydrate 26 g, Dietary Fiber 2 g, Sugars 14 g, Protein 4 g.

LEMON–POPPY SEED ANGEL FOOD CAKE

Makes 12 servings • Serving size: 1 slice

If you like classic angel food cake, leave out the poppy seeds and the lemon zest and substitute vanilla extract for the lemon extract. Any way you make it, angel food cake is just the thing to pair with spring and summer fruits for an easy, elegant finish to any meal.

1 cup cake flour

3/4 cup granular no-calorie sweetener

1/4 cup cornstarch

1 tablespoon poppy seeds

2 teaspoons fresh grated lemon zest

12 large egg whites

1/2 teaspoon cream of tartar

1 teaspoon lemon extract

3/4 cup granulated sugar

1. Preheat the oven to 350°F.

2. Sift together the flour, no-calorie sweetener, and cornstarch. Stir in the poppy seeds and lemon zest and set aside.

3. Combine the egg whites and cream of tartar in a large bowl. Beat at medium speed until foamy. Beat in the lemon extract. Beat in the sugar, 1 tablespoon at a time, beating at high speed until stiff peaks form.

4. Spoon the flour mixture over the egg white mixture in four additions, gently folding in after each addition. Pour the batter into an ungreased 10-inch tube pan.

5. Bake 20 to 25 minutes or until a wooden toothpick inserted in the center of the cake comes out clean. Invert the cake pan and cool the cake completely. Loosen the cake from the sides of the pan with a thin metal spatula. Invert the cake onto a serving platter. The cake can be stored in an airtight container at room temperature up to 2 days.

Exchanges: 1 1/2 Carbohydrate
Calories 127, Calories from Fat 0, Total Fat 0 g, Saturated Fat 0 g, Cholesterol 0 mg, Sodium 55 mg, Total Carbohydrate 26 g, Dietary Fiber 0 g, Sugars 14 g, Protein 5 g.

Brown Sugar Angel Food Cake with Caramel Sauce

Makes 12 servings • Serving size: 1 slice cake with 2 tablespoons sauce

A sprinkling of spices and brown sugar make this angel food cake
an ideal treat for fall and winter. For variety, serve it with the
Maple–Cider Fruit Compote on page 151 instead of the Caramel Sauce.

Brown Sugar Angel Food Cake

1 cup cake flour

3/4 cup granular no-calorie sweetener

1/2 cup dark brown sugar

1/4 cup cornstarch

1/2 teaspoon ground nutmeg

1/2 teaspoon ground cinnamon

1/2 teaspoon ground allspice

1/4 teaspoon ground cloves

12 egg whites

1/2 teaspoon cream of tartar

1/2 teaspoon almond extract

Caramel Sauce

1 egg yolk

1 1/2 cups 1% low-fat milk

1/4 cup dark brown sugar

1 tablespoon cornstarch

Pinch of salt

1/2 teaspoon vanilla extract

Make Cake

1. Preheat the oven to 350°F.

2. Sift together the flour, no-calorie sweetener, brown sugar, cornstarch, nutmeg, cinnamon, allspice, and cloves and set aside.

3. Combine the egg whites and cream of tartar in a large bowl. Beat at medium speed until foamy. Beat in the almond extract and beat at high speed until stiff peaks form.

4. Spoon the flour mixture over the egg white mixture in four additions, gently folding in after each addition. Pour the batter into an ungreased 10-inch tube pan.

5. Bake 20 to 25 minutes or until a wooden toothpick inserted in the center of the cake comes out clean. Invert the cake pan and cool the cake completely.

6. Loosen the cake from sides of pan with a thin metal spatula. Invert the cake onto a serving platter and serve with the Caramel Sauce. The cake can be covered in an airtight container and stored at room temperature up to 2 days.

Make Sauce

1. Place the egg yolk in a medium bowl and set aside.

2. Combine the milk, brown sugar, cornstarch, and salt in a medium saucepan and whisk until smooth. Cook over medium heat until bubbles form around edge of milk mixture.

3. Slowly whisk about 1/3 cup of milk mixture into the egg yolk. Whisk the egg yolk mixture into the milk mixture remaining in the saucepan and cook, stirring constantly (do not whisk) until mixture comes to a boil and thickens. Remove from heat and strain through a fine wire mesh strainer into a bowl. Cool and stir in vanilla.

4. The Caramel Sauce can be covered in an airtight container and stored refrigerated up to 2 days. Bring to room temperature before serving.

Exchanges: 2 Carbohydrate
Calories 149, Calories from Fat 8, Total Fat 1 g, Saturated Fat 0 g, Cholesterol 20 mg, Sodium 89 mg, Total Carbohydrate 29 g, Dietary Fiber 0 g, Sugars 17 g, Protein 6 g.

STRAWBERRY JELLY ROLL CAKE

Makes 10 servings • Serving size: 1 (1-inch) slice cake with 1/4 cup strawberries

Don't be intimidated by making a jelly roll—the trick is to roll it up while it's hot.
After you fill it and reroll it, the cake won't crack and it stays rolled.
Don't tell your guests how easy it is to make!

2/3 cup all-purpose flour

1 teaspoon baking powder

1/4 teaspoon salt

4 large eggs, separated

1/2 cup granulated sugar, divided use

1/3 cup granular no-calorie sweetener

1 tablespoon canola oil

1 teaspoon vanilla extract

1 tablespoon plus 1 teaspoon confectioners' sugar

1 (12-ounce) jar strawberry reduced-sugar preserves, at room temperature

2 1/2 cups sliced fresh strawberries

1. Preheat the oven to 350°F. Line the bottom of a 15 × 10-inch jelly roll pan with parchment paper. Coat the paper and sides of pan with cooking spray. Set aside.

2. Combine the flour, baking powder, and salt in a small bowl and whisk to mix well. Set aside.

3. Place the egg yolks in a large bowl and beat at medium speed until thickened. Gradually beat in 1/4 cup of the sugar and the no-calorie sweetener. Beat in the oil and vanilla. Set aside.

4. Beat the egg whites at high speed until foamy. Gradually beat in the remaining 1/4 cup sugar, beating until stiff peaks form. Gently fold the egg white mixture into the egg yolk mixture. Add the flour mixture to the egg mixture and stir until smooth.

5. Spread the batter evenly into the prepared pan. Bake 10 minutes or until the cake is lightly browned.

6. While the cake bakes, spread a large thin linen or cotton cloth dish towel (not terrycloth) onto the work surface. Sift 1 tablespoon of the confectioners' sugar evenly onto the dish towel.

7. Run a knife along the edge of the cake and turn out onto the sugar-coated dish towel. Remove and discard the parchment paper. Immediately roll up the cake and towel together, starting from the narrow end. Place the rolled cake on a rack, seam side down, and cool completely.

8. Unroll the cake and spread the preserves evenly over the top of the cake. Reroll the cake. Just before serving, place the remaining 1 teaspoon confectioners' sugar in a small fine-mesh sieve and sprinkle over the cake. Serve with berries. The cake is best on the day it is made.

Exchanges: 2 Carbohydrate • 1/2 Fat
Calories 182, Calories from Fat 33, Total Fat 4 g, Saturated Fat 1 g, Cholesterol 85 mg, Sodium 123 mg, Total Carbohydrate 33 g, Dietary Fiber 1 g, Sugars 14 g, Protein 4 g.

Fruit-Filled Layer Cake with White Chocolate Frosting

Makes 12 servings • Serving size: 1 slice

Garnish this lovely layer cake with fresh berries for a special dinner,
or add some candles for a birthday celebration. Make the frosting
before you make the cake, since it has to chill before spreading.

Layer Cake

2 cups cake flour

2 teaspoons baking powder

1 teaspoon baking soda

1/4 teaspoon salt

1/4 cup canola oil

1 large egg

1/3 cup granulated sugar

1/3 cup granular no-calorie sweetener

1 1/3 cups low-fat buttermilk

1 tablespoon vanilla extract

1/2 cup raspberry or strawberry reduced-sugar preserves, at room temperature

White Chocolate Frosting

1/3 cup granulated sugar

1/3 cup granular no-calorie sweetener

1/3 cup all-purpose flour

1 cup fat-free milk

1 1/2 ounces white baking chocolate, chopped

1 teaspoon vanilla extract

Garnish

Fresh raspberries or strawberries (optional)

Make Cake

1. Preheat the oven to 350°F. Coat 2 (8-inch) round cake pans with cooking spray and set aside.

2. Combine the flour, baking powder, baking soda, and salt in a medium bowl and whisk to mix well. Set aside.

3. Combine the oil and egg in a large bowl and beat at medium speed until well mixed. Gradually add the sugar and no-calorie sweetener and beat until mixture is smooth. Add the flour mixture and the buttermilk alternately to the oil mixture, beginning and ending with the flour mixture, beating well after each addition. Beat in the vanilla.

4. Spoon the batter into the prepared pans, smooth the tops, and bake for 15 to 18 minutes or until a wooden toothpick inserted in the center of the cakes comes out clean. Cool the cakes in the pans on wire racks for 10 minutes. Remove the cakes from the pans and cool completely on wire racks.

Make Frosting

1. Combine the sugar, no-calorie sweetener, flour, and milk in a medium saucepan and whisk until the mixture is smooth. Cook over medium heat, whisking constantly, for about 6 minutes or until the mixture comes to a boil and thickens.

2. Remove from the heat and add the chocolate, stirring until the chocolate melts. Spoon the frosting into a medium bowl. Cover and refrigerate 1 hour, stirring occasionally, until cooled and thickened. Stir in the vanilla.

3. Spread the jam between the cake layers. Spread frosting over the top and sides of the cake. Garnish with berries, if desired. The cake can be stored in an airtight container in the refrigerator up to 1 day.

Variation

To use the cake recipe to make Cupcakes with White Chocolate Frosting, line 15 muffin cups with paper liners and coat the liners with cooking spray. Spoon the batter into the prepared cups and bake at 350°F for 12 to 15 minutes or until a wooden toothpick inserted into one of the cupcakes comes out clean. Spread White Chocolate Frosting evenly over the cooled cupcakes.

Exchanges: 2 1/2 Carbohydrate • 1 Fat
Calories 248, Calories from Fat 60, Total Fat 7 g, Saturated Fat 1 g, Cholesterol 20 mg, Sodium 262 mg, Total Carbohydrate 42 g, Dietary Fiber 0 g, Sugars 20 g, Protein 5 g.

CHOCOLATE SOUFFLÉS

Makes 8 servings • Serving size: 1 soufflé

You can make this batter a day ahead, so it's easy to serve these delicious soufflés at your next dinner party.

1/2 cup granulated sugar, divided use

1/2 cup unsweetened cocoa

1/4 cup granular no-calorie sweetener

2 tablespoons all-purpose flour

Pinch of salt

1/2 cup fat-free milk

2 egg yolks

2 teaspoons vanilla extract

4 egg whites

1/8 teaspoon cream of tartar

2 teaspoons confectioners' sugar

1. Combine 1/4 cup of the sugar, the cocoa, no-calorie sweetener, flour, salt, and milk in a medium saucepan and whisk until the mixture is smooth. Cook over medium heat, 3 to 4 minutes, whisking constantly, until the mixture comes to a boil and becomes very thick.

2. Transfer the mixture to a bowl and let stand 5 minutes to cool slightly. Whisk in the egg yolks and vanilla. Cool to room temperature. (You can prepare the recipe up to this point a day ahead and cover and refrigerate the batter. Bring the batter to room temperature before proceeding with the recipe.)

3. Preheat the oven to 350°F. Coat 8 (6-ounce) ramekins or custard cups with cooking spray and set aside.

4. Combine the egg whites and cream of tartar in a large bowl. Beat at high speed until foamy. Gradually beat in the remaining 1/4 cup sugar and beat until stiff peaks form. Fold the egg whites into the chocolate mixture in three additions, mixing until no white streaks remain.

5. Spoon the batter evenly into the prepared ramekins (about 1/3 cup each) and place the ramekins on a baking sheet. Bake 12 to 15 minutes or until the soufflés are puffed and set. Place the confectioners' sugar in a small fine-mesh sieve and sprinkle over the soufflés. Serve immediately.

Exchanges: 1 Carbohydrate • 1/2 Fat
Calories 105, Calories from Fat 18, Total Fat 2 g, Saturated Fat 1 g, Cholesterol 54 mg, Sodium 56 mg, Total Carbohydrate 19 g, Dietary Fiber 2 g, Sugars 15 g, Protein 4 g.

Chocolate Spoon Cake

Makes 9 servings • Serving size: 1/3 cup cake and sauce

Versions of this cake that makes its own sauce abound. This one is a little less sweet and lot lower in calories, but still ooey-gooey good. Make it when there are enough people around to eat it as soon as it comes out of the oven—when the cake cools, it's not nearly as tasty.

1 cup all-purpose flour

1/2 cup plus 3 tablespoons granulated sugar, divided use

1/2 cup granular no-calorie sweetener

1/3 cup plus 3 tablespoons unsweetened cocoa, divided use

2 teaspoons baking powder

1/4 teaspoon salt

1/2 cup 1% low-fat milk

3 tablespoons 67% vegetable oil butter-flavored spread, melted and cooled

2 teaspoons vanilla extract

1 1/2 cups boiling water

1. Preheat the oven to 375°F.

2. Combine the flour, 1/2 cup of the sugar, the no-calorie sweetener, 1/3 cup of the cocoa, the baking powder, and salt in a medium bowl and whisk to mix well. Set aside. Combine the milk, butter-flavored spread, and vanilla in a small bowl and stir to mix well. Add the milk mixture to the flour mixture and stir until smooth. Spread the mixture into an ungreased 1 1/2-quart baking dish.

3. Combine the remaining 3 tablespoons sugar and remaining 3 tablespoons cocoa in a small bowl and stir to mix well. Sprinkle the mixture over the batter in the baking dish. Pour boiling water over the batter (do not stir).

4. Bake 25 to 30 minutes or until the top of the cake develops a cracked surface and the edges are bubbly. Cool in the dish on a wire rack 10 minutes before serving. Serve the cake warm.

Exchanges: 2 Carbohydrate • 1/2 Fat
Calories 164, Calories from Fat 37, Total Fat 4 g, Saturated Fat 1 g, Cholesterol 1 mg, Sodium 185 mg, Total Carbohydrate 31 g, Dietary Fiber 2 g, Sugars 18 g, Protein 3 g.

Quick Breads

Chocolate Chip Banana Bread

Makes 16 servings • Serving size: 1 (1/2-inch) slice

Chocolate chips make this moist bread even more appealing. If chocolate and banana is not your favorite flavor combination, use chopped pecans or walnuts instead of the chocolate.

1 cup all-purpose flour

1 cup whole wheat flour

1/2 cup granular no-calorie sweetener

2 teaspoons baking powder

1/2 teaspoon baking soda

1/4 teaspoon salt

2 cups mashed ripe banana (about 4 medium bananas)

1/2 cup unsweetened applesauce

1/3 cup miniature chocolate chips

1/3 cup canola oil

1/4 cup low-fat buttermilk

1 large egg

1 teaspoon vanilla extract

1. Preheat the oven to 350°F. Coat an 8 × 4-inch loaf pan with cooking spray. Set aside.

2. Combine the all-purpose flour, whole wheat flour, no-calorie sweetener, baking powder, baking soda, and salt in a large bowl and whisk to mix well. Set aside.

3. Combine the banana, applesauce, chocolate chips, oil, buttermilk, egg, and vanilla in a medium bowl and stir to mix well. Add the banana mixture to the flour mixture and stir just until moistened.

4. Spoon the batter into the prepared pan, smooth the top, and bake for 45 to 50 minutes or until a wooden toothpick inserted in the center of the loaf comes out clean.

5. Cool the bread in the pan on a wire rack for 10 minutes. Remove from the pan and cool completely on the wire rack before slicing. The bread can be covered in an airtight container and stored at room temperature up to 3 days.

Exchanges: 1 1/2 Carbohydrate • 1 Fat
Calories 149, Calories from Fat 56, Total Fat 6 g, Saturated Fat 1 g, Cholesterol 13 mg, Sodium 131 mg, Total Carbohydrate 22 g, Dietary Fiber 2 g, Sugars 7 g, Protein 3 g.

FESTIVE CRANBERRY BREAD

Makes 16 servings • Serving size: 1 (1/2-inch) slice

This bright red-speckled bread will make a well-appreciated holiday gift or addition to a brunch menu. Slice any leftovers and warm them in the microwave or toaster oven for a taste as fresh as the day they were baked. If you use frozen cranberries, do not thaw them before chopping.

1 1/2 cups all-purpose flour

1/2 cup whole wheat flour

3/4 cup granulated sugar

1 1/2 teaspoons baking powder

1/2 teaspoon baking soda

1/2 teaspoon salt

1/3 cup 67% vegetable oil butter-flavored spread, chilled

1 1/2 cups fresh cranberries or frozen unthawed cranberries

1 cup low-fat buttermilk

1 large egg

1 tablespoon fresh grated orange zest

1. Preheat the oven to 350°F. Coat an 8 × 4-inch loaf pan with cooking spray and set aside.
2. Place the all-purpose flour, whole wheat flour, sugar, baking powder, baking soda, salt, and butter-flavored spread in a food processor and pulse until spread is uniformly incorporated into the dry ingredients. Transfer the mixture to a large bowl. Do not clean the food processor.
3. Place the cranberries in the food processor and pulse until coarsely chopped, then transfer to a medium bowl. Add the buttermilk, egg, and orange zest to the cranberries and stir until well combined. Add the cranberry mixture to the flour mixture and stir just until moistened.
4. Spoon into the prepared pan, smooth the top of the batter, and bake 35 to 40 minutes or until a wooden toothpick inserted in the center of the loaf comes out clean.
5. Cool the bread in the pan on a wire rack for 10 minutes. Remove from the pan and cool completely on the wire rack before slicing. The bread can be covered in an airtight container and stored at room temperature up to 3 days or frozen up to 2 months.

Exchanges: 1 1/2 Carbohydrate • 1/2 Fat
Calories 135, Calories from Fat 34, Total Fat 4 g, Saturated Fat 1 g, Cholesterol 14 mg, Sodium 197 mg, Total Carbohydrate 23 g, Dietary Fiber 1 g, Sugars 11 g, Protein 3 g.

Apple–Walnut Sweet Bread

Makes 16 servings • Serving size: 1 (1/2-inch) slice

Moist and lightly spiced, this loaf is like having a slice of fall on your plate.
Enjoy it on a picnic or with a cup of tea in the backyard.

1 cup all-purpose flour

3/4 cup whole wheat flour

3/4 cup light brown sugar

2 teaspoons ground cinnamon

1 teaspoon baking powder

1/4 teaspoon salt

1/3 cup apple cider or
unsweetened apple juice

1/3 cup canola oil

1 large egg

2 medium Granny Smith
apples, peeled and coarsely
shredded (about 1 1/2 cups)

1/2 cup chopped walnuts

1. Preheat the oven to 350°F. Coat an 8 × 4-inch loaf pan with cooking spray and set aside.

2. Combine the all-purpose flour, whole wheat flour, brown sugar, cinnamon, baking powder, and salt in a large bowl and whisk to mix well. Set aside.

3. Combine the apple cider, oil, and egg in a medium bowl and whisk to mix well. Stir in the apples and walnuts. Add the apple cider mixture to the flour mixture and stir just until moistened. (Batter will be very thick.)

4. Spoon the batter into the prepared pan, smooth the top, and bake for 45 to 50 minutes or until a wooden toothpick inserted in the center of the loaf comes out clean.

5. Cool the bread in the pan on a wire rack for 10 minutes. Remove from the pan and cool completely on the wire rack before slicing. The bread can be covered in an airtight container and stored at room temperature up to 3 days.

Exchanges: 1 1/2 Carbohydrate • 1 1/2 Fat
Calories 167, Calories from Fat 67, Total Fat 7 g, Saturated Fat 1 g, Cholesterol 13 mg, Sodium 68 mg, Total Carbohydrate 24 g, Dietary Fiber 2 g, Sugars 13 g, Protein 3 g.

DRIED APRICOT–PEAR LOAF

Makes 16 servings • Serving size: 1 (1/2-inch) slice

For the best flavor, make sure your pear is ripe: it should yield to gentle pressure at the base of the neck and have a fragrant aroma. Dried apricot and fresh pear makes an unusual, but incredibly tasty, pairing in this fruity bread.

1/3 cup walnut pieces
1 cup all-purpose flour
3/4 cup whole wheat flour
1/2 cup light brown sugar
2 teaspoons baking powder
1/2 teaspoon ground cinnamon
1/4 teaspoon ground nutmeg
1/4 teaspoon baking soda
1/4 teaspoon salt
1/3 cup canola oil
1/4 cup low-fat buttermilk
2 large eggs
1 cup dried apricots, chopped
1 ripe pear, peeled and coarsely shredded (about 3/4 cup)

1. Preheat the oven to 350°F. Place the nuts in a small baking pan. Bake, stirring once, 5 to 8 minutes or until the nuts are lightly toasted. Maintain the oven temperature. Set the nuts aside to cool. Finely chop the cooled nuts.

2. Coat an 8 × 4-inch loaf pan with cooking spray. Set aside.

3. Combine the all-purpose flour, whole wheat flour, brown sugar, baking powder, cinnamon, nutmeg, baking soda, and salt in a large bowl and whisk to mix well.

4. Combine the canola oil, buttermilk, and eggs in a medium bowl and whisk to mix well. Add the oil mixture to the flour mixture and stir just until moistened. Gently stir in the apricots, pear, and walnuts.

5. Spoon the batter into the prepared pan, smooth the top, and bake 35 to 40 minutes or until a wooden toothpick inserted in the center of the loaf comes out clean.

6. Cool the bread in the pan on a wire rack for 10 minutes. Remove from the pan and cool completely on the wire rack before slicing. The bread can be stored in an airtight container at room temperature up to 3 days or frozen up to 2 months.

Exchanges: 2 Carbohydrate • 1 Fat
Calories 181, Calories from Fat 63, Total Fat 7 g, Saturated Fat 1 g, Cholesterol 27 mg, Sodium 119 mg, Total Carbohydrate 28 g, Dietary Fiber 2 g, Sugars 16 g, Protein 3 g.

CARROT–ZUCCHINI BREAD

Makes 16 servings • Serving size: 1 (1/2-inch) slice

Pumpkin pie spice adds unexpected flavor to this colorful, healthy loaf.
Don't be tempted to skip the extra step of pressing the zucchini between
layers of paper towels, or the bread will be soggy.

1 1/2 cups coarsely shredded zucchini

1 1/2 cups coarsely shredded carrot

1/3 cup canola oil

1/4 cup low-fat buttermilk

2 large eggs

1 teaspoon vanilla extract

1 cup all-purpose flour

1 cup whole wheat flour

3/4 cup light brown sugar

2 teaspoons baking powder

1 1/2 teaspoons pumpkin pie spice

1/4 teaspoon salt

1. Preheat the oven to 350°F. Coat an 8 × 4-inch loaf pan with cooking spray and set aside.

2. Spread the zucchini onto several thicknesses of paper towels, cover with additional layers of paper towels, roll up jellyroll fashion, and press to remove excess liquid. Let stand 5 minutes, pressing occasionally. Place the zucchini and carrot in a medium bowl.

3. Combine the oil, buttermilk, eggs, and vanilla in a small bowl, whisk until smooth, and stir into the zucchini mixture. Set aside.

4. Combine the all-purpose flour, whole wheat flour, brown sugar, baking powder, pumpkin pie spice, and salt in a large bowl and whisk to mix well. Add the zucchini mixture to the flour mixture and stir just until moistened. (The batter will be very thick.)

5. Spoon the batter into the prepared pan, smooth the top, and bake 45 to 50 minutes or until a wooden toothpick inserted in the center of the loaf comes out clean.

6. Cool the bread in the pan on a wire rack for 10 minutes. Remove from the pan and cool completely on the wire rack before slicing. The bread can be covered in an airtight container and stored at room temperature up to 3 days.

Exchanges: 1 1/2 Carbohydrate • 1 Fat
Calories 152, Calories from Fat 49, Total Fat 5 g, Saturated Fat 1 g, Cholesterol 27 mg, Sodium 109 mg, Total Carbohydrate 24 g, Dietary Fiber 2 g, Sugars 11 g, Protein 3 g.

Hummingbird Loaf Cake

Makes 16 servings • Serving size: 1 (1/2-inch) slice

This is the classic pineapple, banana, and pecan cake, lower in calories with
less oil, nuts, and sugar, and healthier with part whole wheat flour instead of all white.
You won't even miss the cream cheese frosting!

1 cup all-purpose flour

1/2 cup whole wheat flour

3/4 cup granulated sugar

1/2 teaspoon baking soda

1/2 teaspoon ground
cinnamon

1/4 teaspoon salt

1 (8-ounce) can crushed
pineapple in juice

1/3 cup canola oil

1 large egg

1 teaspoon vanilla extract

1 cup mashed ripe banana
(about 2 medium bananas)

1/3 cup chopped pecans

1. Preheat the oven to 350°F. Coat an 8 × 4-inch loaf pan
   with cooking spray and set aside.

2. Combine the all-purpose flour, whole wheat flour, sugar,
   baking soda, cinnamon, and salt in a large bowl and whisk
   to mix well. Set aside.

3. Place the pineapple in a wire sieve and press with a spatula
   to remove as much liquid as possible. Place the pineapple
   in a medium bowl and add the oil, egg, and vanilla. Stir to
   mix well. Stir in the banana and pecans. Add the pineapple
   mixture to the flour mixture and stir just until moistened.

4. Spoon the batter into prepared pan, smooth the top, and
   bake for 40 to 45 minutes or until a wooden toothpick
   inserted in the center of the loaf comes out clean.

5. Cool the cake in the pan on a wire rack for 10 minutes.
   Remove from the pan and cool completely on the wire
   rack before slicing. The cake can be covered in an airtight
   container and stored at room temperature up to 3 days.

Exchanges: 1 1/2 Carbohydrate • 1 Fat
Calories 158, Calories from Fat 60, Total Fat 7 g, Saturated Fat 1 g, Cholesterol 13 mg,
Sodium 81 mg, Total Carbohydrate 23 g, Dietary Fiber 1 g, Sugars 13 g, Protein 2 g.

GOLDEN OATMEAL–WHEAT LOAVES

Makes 14 servings • Serving size: 1 (3/4-inch) slice

Spread this tasty bread with jam at breakfast or snack time, or serve it with soup for a nourishing lunch. The diminutive loaves make a thoughtful gift with an accompanying jar of homemade jam. Toasted slices are delicious spread with natural peanut butter.

2 cups all-purpose flour

1 cup whole wheat flour

1 1/2 teaspoons salt

1 teaspoon baking soda

1 teaspoon baking powder

1 cup plus 1 tablespoon old-fashioned (not quick-cooking) oats, divided use

2 cups low-fat buttermilk

2 tablespoons canola oil

2 tablespoons molasses

1. Preheat the oven to 350°F. Coat 2 (5 1/2 × 3-inch) loaf pans with cooking spray and set aside.
2. Combine the all-purpose flour, whole wheat flour, salt, baking soda, and baking powder in a large bowl and whisk to mix well. Stir in 1 cup of the oats and set aside.
3. Combine the buttermilk, canola oil, and molasses in a medium bowl and whisk until the mixture is smooth. Add the buttermilk mixture to the flour mixture and stir until a stiff dough forms.
4. Transfer the dough to a lightly floured surface, sprinkle lightly with flour, and using floured hands, knead 1 minute or until the dough is smooth.
5. Divide the dough in half and place in the prepared pans. Sprinkle the tops of the loaves evenly with the remaining 1 tablespoon oats. Bake for 30 to 35 minutes or until the tops of the loaves are lightly browned.
6. Cool the bread in the pans on a wire rack for 10 minutes. Remove from the pans and cool completely on the wire rack. Serve warm or at room temperature. The bread can be stored in an airtight container at room temperature up to 2 days.

Exchanges: 2 Starch

Calories 157, Calories from Fat 27, Total Fat 3 g, Saturated Fat 1 g, Cholesterol 1 mg, Sodium 404 mg, Total Carbohydrate 28 g, Dietary Fiber 2 g, Sugars 4 g, Protein 5 g.

DAINTY DRIED FRUIT LOAVES

Makes 28 servings • Serving size: 1 (3/4-inch) slice

Slice these adorable little loaves and serve with tea, or give them
as an especially nice holiday gift.

2 1/2 cups all-purpose flour

1 teaspoon baking powder

1 teaspoon baking soda

1/4 teaspoon salt

1 tablespoon fresh grated
orange zest

1 1/4 cups fresh-squeezed
orange juice

3/4 cup granulated sugar

1/3 cup canola oil

1 large egg

1 teaspoon vanilla extract

1/2 cup golden raisins

1/2 cup dried cranberries

1/2 cup chopped pecans

1/4 cup dried currants

1. Preheat the oven to 350°F. Coat 4 (5 1/2 × 3-inch) loaf pans with cooking spray and set aside.

2. Combine the flour, baking powder, baking soda, and salt in a medium bowl, whisk to mix well, and set aside. Combine the orange zest and orange juice in a small bowl and set aside.

3. Combine the sugar, oil, and egg in a large bowl and beat at medium speed for 1 minute or until mixture is pale in color. Add the flour mixture and orange juice mixture alternately to the sugar mixture, beginning and ending with the flour mixture, beating well after each addition. Beat in the vanilla. Stir in the raisins, cranberries, pecans, and currants.

4. Spoon the batter evenly into the prepared pans and bake 25 to 30 minutes or until a wooden toothpick inserted in the centers of the loaves comes out clean.

5. Cool the loaves in the pans on a wire rack for 5 minutes. Remove from the pans and cool completely on the wire rack. The loaves can be covered in an airtight container and stored at room temperature up to 3 days.

Exchanges: 1 1/2 Carbohydrate • 1/2 Fat
Calories 126, Calories from Fat 40, Total Fat 4 g, Saturated Fat 0 g, Cholesterol 8 mg,
Sodium 82 mg, Total Carbohydrate 20 g, Dietary Fiber 1 g, Sugars 11 g, Protein 2 g.

JEWELED SODA BREAD

Makes 12 servings • Serving size: 1 slice

How can a few simple ingredients create such a delicious bread? A colorful mix of dried fruits plays off the hearty whole grains for an unbeatable flavor.

1/2 cup orange juice

1/2 cup golden raisins

1/2 cup chopped dried apricots

1/4 cup dried currants

2 cups whole wheat flour

1 1/2 cups all-purpose flour

1 cup unprocessed wheat bran

1/4 cup fat-free instant dry milk

1 tablespoon light brown sugar

1 1/2 teaspoons salt

1 teaspoon baking soda

1/2 teaspoon cream of tartar

1/4 cup 67% vegetable oil butter-flavored spread, chilled

2 cups low-fat buttermilk

1. Preheat the oven to 375°F. Coat a 9-inch round cake pan with cooking spray and set aside.

2. Place the orange juice in a small saucepan and heat over medium heat until hot but not boiling. Remove from the heat and add the raisins, apricots, and currants. Cover and let stand 10 minutes or until most of the juice is absorbed.

3. Combine the whole wheat flour, all-purpose flour, bran, fat-free dry milk, brown sugar, salt, baking soda, and cream of tartar in a large bowl. Add the butter-flavored spread and blend into dry ingredients using a pastry blender or your fingertips until the spread is uniformly incorporated.

4. Add the buttermilk and the reserved fruit mixture and stir until a sticky dough forms. Transfer the dough to a lightly floured surface, sprinkle lightly with flour, and using floured hands, knead 2 minutes until the dough is smooth.

5. Place the dough in the prepared pan and bake 30 to 35 minutes or until the top is lightly browned and the loaf sounds hollow when tapped.

6. Cool the loaf in the pan on a wire rack for 10 minutes. Remove from the pan and cool completely on the wire rack before slicing. The bread can be covered in an airtight container and stored at room temperature up to 3 days.

Exchanges: 3 Carbohydrate • 1/2 Fat
Calories 246, Calories from Fat 39, Total Fat 4 g, Saturated Fat 1 g, Cholesterol 2 mg, Sodium 481 mg, Total Carbohydrate 48 g, Dietary Fiber 6 g, Sugars 17 g, Protein 8 g.

ORANGE–ALMOND TEA CAKE

Makes 8 servings • Serving size: 1 slice

Take care to process the almonds until they are very finely ground so the cake will have a delicate texture. Serve slices with fresh berries for an understated, yet elegant, dessert.

3/4 cup slivered almonds

1/2 cup granulated sugar

1/4 cup granular no-calorie sweetener

1 1/2 cups all-purpose flour

1/4 teaspoon salt

1/3 cup canola oil

1 tablespoon fresh grated orange zest

1 cup fresh-squeezed orange juice

1 teaspoon almond extract

6 egg whites

1 teaspoon confectioners' sugar

1. Preheat the oven to 350°F. Coat an 8-inch round cake pan with cooking spray and set aside.

2. Combine the almonds, sugar, and no-calorie sweetener in a food processor and process for 1 minute or until nuts are finely ground. Transfer the mixture to a large bowl and stir in the flour and salt.

3. Combine the oil, orange zest, orange juice, and almond extract in a medium bowl and stir to mix well. Add the oil mixture to the almond mixture and stir to mix well.

4. Place the egg whites in a large bowl and beat at high speed until stiff peaks form. Add the egg whites to the almond mixture in two additions, mixing until no white streaks remain. Pour the batter into the prepared pan and bake 30 to 35 minutes or until a wooden toothpick inserted in the center of the cake comes out clean and the edge of the cake is very lightly browned.

5. Cool the cake in the pan on a wire rack for 10 minutes. Remove from the pan and cool completely on the wire rack.

6. Just before serving, place the confectioners' sugar in a small fine-mesh sieve and sprinkle over the cake. The cake can be stored in an airtight container at room temperature up to 2 days.

Exchanges: 2 1/2 Carbohydrate • 2 1/2 Fat
Calories 310, Calories from Fat 134, Total Fat 15 g, Saturated Fat 1 g, Cholesterol 0 mg, Sodium 114 mg, Total Carbohydrate 37 g, Dietary Fiber 2 g, Sugars 18 g, Protein 8 g.

DEVIL'S FOOD SNACK CAKE

Makes 9 servings • Serving size: 1 (3-inch) square

This simple, rich, and chocolaty cake calls out for a glass of cold milk. Serve it plain for an afternoon treat, or dress it up for company with frozen yogurt and a garnish of fresh fruit.

3/4 cup all-purpose flour

1/2 cup unsweetened cocoa

3/4 teaspoon baking powder

1/4 teaspoon baking soda

1/4 teaspoon salt

1/2 cup granulated sugar

1/2 cup granular no-calorie sweetener

1/3 cup low-fat buttermilk

3 tablespoons canola oil

2 large eggs

2 teaspoons vanilla extract

1 teaspoon confectioners' sugar

1. Preheat the oven to 350°F. Coat an 8 × 8-inch baking pan with cooking spray and set aside.

2. Combine the flour, cocoa, baking powder, baking soda, and salt in a medium bowl and whisk to mix well. Set aside.

3. Combine the sugar, no-calorie sweetener, buttermilk, oil, and eggs in a large bowl. Beat at medium speed for 2 minutes or until mixture is smooth and light in color. Beat in the vanilla. Add the flour mixture and beat at low speed just until blended.

4. Pour the batter into the prepared pan. Bake 15 minutes or until a wooden toothpick inserted in the center of the cake comes out clean.

5. Cool the cake in the pan on a wire rack for 10 minutes. Remove from the pan and cool completely on the wire rack. Just before serving, place the confectioners' sugar in a small fine-mesh sieve and sprinkle over the cake. The cake can be covered in an airtight container and stored at room temperature up to 3 days.

Exchanges: 1 1/2 Carbohydrate • 1 Fat
Calories 162, Calories from Fat 59, Total Fat 7 g, Saturated Fat 1 g, Cholesterol 47 mg, Sodium 156 mg, Total Carbohydrate 24 g, Dietary Fiber 2 g, Sugars 14 g, Protein 4 g.

LEMON-GLAZED BLUEBERRY–CORNMEAL COFFEE CAKE

Makes 8 servings • Serving size: 1 slice

Cornmeal imparts a terrific texture to this cake, and buttermilk gives it melt-in-your-mouth tenderness. A drizzle of lemon glaze adds sweetness without a lot of additional sugar.

1 cup all-purpose flour

1/4 cup yellow cornmeal (not cornmeal mix)

1 teaspoon baking powder

1/2 teaspoon baking soda

1/4 teaspoon salt

1/3 cup granulated sugar

3 tablespoons 67% vegetable oil butter-flavored spread, at room temperature

1 large egg

1 tablespoon fresh grated lemon zest

3/4 cup low-fat buttermilk

1 cup fresh blueberries or frozen unthawed blueberries

1/3 cup confectioners' sugar

2 to 3 teaspoons fresh lemon juice

1. Preheat the oven to 350°F. Coat an 8-inch round cake pan with cooking spray and set aside.

2. Combine the flour, cornmeal, baking powder, baking soda, and salt in a medium bowl and whisk to mix well. Set aside.

3. Combine the sugar and butter-flavored spread in a large bowl and beat at medium speed until the mixture is light and fluffy. Beat in the egg and lemon zest. Add the flour mixture to the sugar mixture, alternating with the buttermilk, beginning and ending with the flour mixture. Gently stir in the blueberries.

4. Spoon the batter into prepared pan. Bake 25 to 30 minutes or until a wooden toothpick inserted in the center of the cake comes out clean.

5. Cool the cake in the pan on wire rack for 10 minutes. Remove from the pan and place the cake on the wire rack. Place the rack on waxed paper.

6. Combine the confectioners' sugar and 2 teaspoons of the lemon juice in a small bowl, stirring until well mixed. Stir in additional lemon juice, a few drops at a time, until the desired drizzling consistency is reached. Drizzle over the warm cake. Serve the cake warm or at room temperature. The cake is best on the day it is made.

Exchanges: 2 Carbohydrate • 1 Fat
Calories 186, Calories from Fat 42, Total Fat 5 g, Saturated Fat 1 g, Cholesterol 27 mg, Sodium 264 mg, Total Carbohydrate 33 g, Dietary Fiber 1 g, Sugars 16 g, Protein 4 g.

RASPBERRY–BROWN SUGAR CRUMB CAKE

Makes 15 servings • Serving size: 1 (3 × 2 1/2-inch) piece

Perfect for a potluck, brunch, or tea, this cake is a guaranteed crowd-pleaser. It's a tangy yogurt cake, loaded with berries and sprinkled with a crunchy brown sugar topping—what's not to love!

3 cups all-purpose flour

1/2 cup granulated sugar

1/2 cup granular no-calorie sweetener

2 teaspoons baking powder

1/2 teaspoon baking soda

1/4 teaspoon salt

6 tablespoons 67% vegetable oil butter-flavored spread, chilled, divided use

2 tablespoons light brown sugar

2 large eggs

1 3/4 cups plain fat-free yogurt

2 teaspoons vanilla extract

3 cups fresh raspberries or blueberries or 1 (12-ounce) package frozen unthawed raspberries or blueberries

1. Preheat the oven to 375°F. Coat a 13 x 9-inch baking pan with cooking spray and set aside.

2. Combine the flour, granulated sugar, no-calorie sweetener, baking powder, baking soda, and salt in a large bowl. Add 4 tablespoons of the butter-flavored spread and blend into dry ingredients using a pastry blender or your fingertips until the spread is uniformly incorporated.

3. To make the crumb topping, transfer 1/2 cup of the flour mixture to a small bowl. Add the remaining 2 tablespoons of the butter-flavored spread and the brown sugar. Blend in using a pastry blender or your fingertips until the spread and sugar are uniformly incorporated. Set the crumb topping aside.

4. Combine the eggs, yogurt, and vanilla in a medium bowl and whisk until smooth. Add the egg mixture to the first flour mixture and stir just until combined. Gently stir in the berries.

5. Spread the batter into the prepared pan and sprinkle evenly with the crumb topping. Bake 25 minutes or until the edges of cake are browned and a wooden toothpick inserted in the center of the cake comes out clean.

6. Cool the cake completely in the pan on a wire rack before cutting. The cake is best on the day it is made.

Exchanges: 2 Carbohydrate • 1 Fat
Calories 198, Calories from Fat 44, Total Fat 5 g, Saturated Fat 1 g, Cholesterol 30 mg, Sodium 195 mg, Total Carbohydrate 33 g, Dietary Fiber 2 g, Sugars 13 g, Protein 5 g.

MAPLE-GLAZED PUMPKIN–WALNUT MUFFINS

Makes 12 servings • Serving size: 1 muffin

Keep a stash of these in the freezer and reheat in the microwave for breakfast on the go. Brushing the tops with real maple syrup (pancake syrup will do in a pinch) adds moisture and gives them a unique sweet flavor.

1/3 cup chopped walnuts

3/4 cup all-purpose flour

3/4 cup whole wheat flour

1/2 cup light brown sugar

2 teaspoons baking powder

2 teaspoons pumpkin pie spice

1/2 teaspoon baking soda

1/4 teaspoon salt

1 cup solid-pack pumpkin (not pumpkin pie filling)

1/3 cup plain low-fat yogurt

1/4 cup canola oil

1 large egg

1 teaspoon vanilla extract

1 tablespoon maple syrup

1. Preheat the oven to 350°F. Line 12 muffin cups with paper liners and coat the liners with cooking spray. Set aside.

2. Place the walnuts in a small baking pan and bake, stirring once, until lightly toasted, 5 to 8 minutes. Set aside to cool. Maintain the oven temperature.

3. Combine the all-purpose flour, whole wheat flour, brown sugar, baking powder, pumpkin pie spice, baking soda, and salt in a large bowl and whisk to mix well.

4. Combine the pumpkin, yogurt, oil, egg, and vanilla in a medium bowl and whisk until smooth. Add the pumpkin mixture and walnuts to the flour mixture and stir just until moistened. Spoon the batter evenly into the prepared muffin liners and bake 15 to 17 minutes or until the tops of the muffins are lightly browned.

5. Immediately brush the tops of the muffins with maple syrup. Cool the muffins in the pan on a wire rack for 5 minutes. Remove from the pan and cool completely on the wire rack. Serve the muffins warm or at room temperature. The muffins can be stored in an airtight container at room temperature up to 2 days or frozen up to 2 months.

Exchanges: 1 1/2 Carbohydrate • 1 1/2 Fat
Calories 174, Calories from Fat 68, Total Fat 8 g, Saturated Fat 1 g, Cholesterol 18 mg, Sodium 177 mg, Total Carbohydrate 24 g, Dietary Fiber 2 g, Sugars 11 g, Protein 3 g.

LEMON SURPRISE MUFFINS

Makes 12 servings • Serving size: 1 muffin

For variety, use any flavor of fruit spread or preserves that you have on hand to fill these tender muffins. A tiny bit of sugar sprinkled on the top gives them extra sweetness and crunch.

1 3/4 cups all-purpose flour

1/3 cup plus 1 tablespoon granulated sugar, divided use

1 1/2 teaspoons baking powder

1/2 teaspoon baking soda

1/4 teaspoon salt

1 cup plain low-fat yogurt

2 tablespoons canola oil

1 large egg

1 tablespoon fresh grated lemon zest

1/4 cup natural fruit spread or reduced-sugar preserves

1. Preheat the oven to 350°F. Line 12 muffin cups with paper liners and coat the liners with cooking spray. Set aside.

2. Combine the flour, 1/3 cup of the sugar, baking powder, baking soda, and salt in a large bowl and whisk to mix well. Set aside.

3. Combine the yogurt, oil, egg, and lemon zest in a small bowl and whisk until smooth. Add the yogurt mixture to the flour mixture and stir just until moistened.

4. Spoon 1 rounded tablespoon of the batter into each of the prepared muffin liners and spread the batter to cover the bottom of the liners. Spoon 1 level teaspoon of the fruit spread into the centers of the batter. Top evenly with the remaining batter and spread the batter to cover the fruit spread. Sprinkle the tops evenly with the remaining 1 tablespoon sugar. Bake for 15 to 18 minutes or until the tops of the muffins are lightly browned.

5. Cool in the pan on a wire rack for 5 minutes. Remove from the pan and cool completely on the wire rack. Serve the muffins warm or at room temperature. The muffins are best on the day they are made.

Exchanges: 1 1/2 Carbohydrate • 1/2 Fat
Calories 145, Calories from Fat 29, Total Fat 3 g, Saturated Fat 1 g, Cholesterol 19 mg, Sodium 167 mg, Total Carbohydrate 25 g, Dietary Fiber 1 g, Sugars 11 g, Protein 3 g.

Berry Bran Muffins

Makes 12 servings • Serving size: 1 muffin

Scrumptious berries give these muffins such a big dose of flavor that even kids will eat them. With 4 grams of fiber in each one, they're a healthful way to greet the day.

1 cup unprocessed wheat bran

1 cup whole wheat flour

1/4 cup light brown sugar

1 teaspoon baking soda

1/4 teaspoon salt

1 cup low-fat buttermilk

1/4 cup unsweetened applesauce

3 tablespoons canola oil

1 large egg

1 teaspoon vanilla extract

1 cup fresh blueberries, raspberries, or cranberries (or substitute frozen, unthawed berries)

1. Preheat the oven to 350°F. Line 12 muffin cups with paper liners and coat the liners with cooking spray. Set aside.

2. Combine the bran, flour, brown sugar, baking soda, and salt in a large bowl. Set aside.

3. Combine the buttermilk, applesauce, oil, egg, and vanilla in a medium bowl and whisk to mix well. Add the buttermilk mixture to the bran mixture and stir just until the batter is moistened. Gently stir in the berries.

4. Spoon the batter evenly into the prepared muffin liners and bake 15 to 17 minutes or until the tops of the muffins are lightly browned.

5. Cool the muffins in the pan on a wire rack for 5 minutes. Remove from the pan and cool completely on the wire rack. Serve the muffins warm or at room temperature. The muffins can be covered in an airtight container and stored at room temperature up to 3 days or frozen up to 2 months.

Exchanges: 1 Carbohydrate • 1 Fat

Calories 117, Calories from Fat 41, Total Fat 5 g, Saturated Fat 1 g, Cholesterol 18 mg, Sodium 183 mg, Total Carbohydrate 18 g, Dietary Fiber 4 g, Sugars 7 g, Protein 3 g.

WHOLE WHEAT HONEY MUFFINS

Makes 12 servings • Serving size: 1 muffin

Shredded apple and prune puree make these muffins super-moist. Store them in the refrigerator and they will keep for a week—just pop one in the microwave, grab a cup of coffee, and you're ready for breakfast on the run.

1 3/4 cups whole wheat flour

1/4 cup fat-free instant dry milk

2 teaspoons baking powder

1/2 teaspoon baking soda

1/4 teaspoon salt

3/4 cup low-fat buttermilk

1/2 cup honey

1/3 cup prune puree

1 large egg

1 medium Granny Smith apple, peeled and coarsely shredded (about 3/4 cup)

1 tablespoon fresh grated orange zest

1. Preheat the oven to 350°F. Line 12 muffin cups with paper liners and coat the liners with cooking spray. Set aside.

2. Combine the flour, fat-free dry milk, baking powder, baking soda, and salt in a large bowl and whisk to mix well. Set aside.

3. Combine the buttermilk, honey, prune puree, and egg in a medium bowl and whisk until smooth. Stir in the apple and orange zest. Add the buttermilk mixture to the flour mixture and stir just until moistened.

4. Spoon the batter evenly into the prepared muffin liners and bake for 15 minutes or until the muffins are lightly browned.

5. Cool the muffins in the pan on a wire rack for 5 minutes. Remove from the pan and cool completely on the wire rack. Serve the muffins warm or at room temperature. The muffins can be covered in an airtight container and stored at room temperature up to 3 days or frozen up to 2 months.

Exchanges: 2 Carbohydrate
Calories 150, Calories from Fat 8, Total Fat 1 g, Saturated Fat 0 g, Cholesterol 18 mg, Sodium 195 mg, Total Carbohydrate 34 g, Dietary Fiber 3 g, Sugars 18 g, Protein 4 g.

Tropical Blueberry Muffins

Makes 12 servings • Serving size: 1 muffin

Loaded with flavor from fresh lime zest and ground ginger, these blueberry muffins will make supermarket versions taste humdrum in comparison. And blueberries are packed with disease-fighting antioxidants—as if you needed another reason to try these!

2 cups all-purpose flour

1/4 cup granulated sugar

1/4 cup granular no-calorie sweetener

1 teaspoon baking powder

3/4 teaspoon ground ginger

1/2 teaspoon baking soda

1/4 teaspoon salt

1 1/4 cups low-fat buttermilk

1/4 cup canola oil

1 large egg

1 tablespoon fresh grated lime zest

1 cup fresh blueberries or frozen unthawed blueberries

1. Preheat the oven to 350°F. Line 12 muffin cups with paper liners and coat the liners with cooking spray. Set aside.

2. Combine the flour, sugar, no-calorie sweetener, baking powder, ginger, baking soda, and salt in a large bowl and whisk to mix well.

3. Combine the buttermilk, oil, egg, and lime zest in a medium bowl and whisk to mix well. Add the buttermilk mixture to the flour mixture and stir just until moistened. Gently stir in the blueberries. Spoon the batter evenly into the prepared muffin liners and bake 15 to 18 minutes or until the tops of the muffins are lightly browned.

4. Cool the muffins in the pan on a wire rack for 5 minutes. Remove from the pan and cool completely on the wire rack. Serve the muffins warm or at room temperature. The muffins can be covered in an airtight container and stored at room temperature up to 2 days.

Exchanges: 1 1/2 Carbohydrate • 1 Fat
Calories 158, Calories from Fat 49, Total Fat 5 g, Saturated Fat 1 g, Cholesterol 19 mg, Sodium 164 mg, Total Carbohydrate 24 g, Dietary Fiber 1 g, Sugars 7 g, Protein 4 g.

CORNMEAL–ZUCCHINI MUFFINS

Makes 12 servings • Serving size: 1 muffin

Shredded zucchini keeps these muffins moist and cornmeal gives them a hearty texture.
They're not too sweet, so enjoy them at brunch, for an afternoon snack,
or served with a bowl of soup for lunch.

1 cup all-purpose flour

1 cup yellow cornmeal
(not cornmeal mix)

1 teaspoon baking powder

1/2 teaspoon baking soda

1/4 teaspoon salt

1 cup low-fat buttermilk

1/4 cup canola oil

1/4 cup honey

1 large egg

1 cup shredded zucchini

1. Preheat the oven to 350°F. Line 12 muffin cups with paper liners and coat the liners with cooking spray. Set aside.

2. Combine the flour, cornmeal, baking powder, baking soda, and salt in a large bowl and whisk to mix well.

3. Combine the buttermilk, oil, honey, and egg in a medium bowl and whisk to mix well. Stir in the zucchini. Add the buttermilk mixture to the flour mixture and stir just until moistened. Spoon the batter evenly into the prepared muffin liners and bake 15 to 18 minutes or until the tops of the muffins are lightly browned.

4. Cool the muffins in the pan on a wire rack for 5 minutes. Remove from the pan and cool on the wire rack. Serve the muffins warm or at room temperature. The muffins can be covered in an airtight container and stored at room temperature up to 2 days.

Exchanges: 1 1/2 Carbohydrate • 1 Fat
Calories 158, Calories from Fat 49, Total Fat 5 g, Saturated Fat 1 g, Cholesterol 18 mg, Sodium 160 mg, Total Carbohydrate 24 g, Dietary Fiber 1 g, Sugars 7 g, Protein 3 g.

PEACH MELBA SHORTCAKES

Makes 8 servings • Serving size: 1 biscuit with 1/4 cup peaches and 2 tablespoons sauce

A variation on the traditional strawberry shortcake, this is an easy version to make. Shape the dough into rounds with your hands and you don't even have to get out the rolling pin. Try them with strawberries instead of peaches, too.

Biscuits

1/3 cup low-fat buttermilk

1/2 teaspoon vanilla extract

1 cup all-purpose flour

2 1/2 tablespoons granulated sugar, divided use

1 teaspoon baking powder

1/4 teaspoon baking soda

1/4 teaspoon salt

3 tablespoons 67% vegetable oil butter-flavored spread, chilled

Raspberry Sauce

1 (12-ounce) package frozen unsweetened raspberries, thawed

2 tablespoons granulated sugar

1 tablespoon fresh lemon juice

Filling

4 medium peaches peeled, pitted, and sliced (about 2 cups)

Make Biscuits

1. Preheat the oven to 375°F. Coat a baking sheet with cooking spray and set aside.

2. Combine the buttermilk and vanilla in a small bowl. Set aside. Combine the flour, 2 tablespoons of the sugar, the baking powder, baking soda, salt, and butter-flavored spread in a food processor and pulse until the spread is uniformly incorporated into the dry ingredients. Transfer the mixture to a large bowl. Add the buttermilk mixture and stir just until moistened.

3. Using floured hands, shape the dough into 8 (2-inch) diameter rounds and place on the prepared pan, spacing about 1/2-inch apart. Sprinkle evenly with the remaining 1/2 tablespoon sugar. Bake 10 to 12 minutes, or until the tops of the biscuits are lightly browned. Transfer to a wire rack. Serve the biscuits warm or at room temperature.

Make Sauce

1. Combine the raspberries, sugar, and lemon juice in a food processor or blender and puree. Press mixture through a fine wire mesh sieve, discarding solids.

2. To serve, split the biscuits in half horizontally. Place the bottom halves in each of 8 shallow serving dishes. Top each with 1/4 cup of the peaches. Top the peaches with the top halves of the biscuits. Drizzle each one with 2 tablespoons of the sauce. Serve immediately.

Exchanges: 2 Carbohydrate • 1/2 Fat
Calories 154, Calories from Fat 35, Total Fat 4 g, Saturated Fat 1 g, Cholesterol 0 mg, Sodium 203 mg, Total Carbohydrate 28 g, Dietary Fiber 1 g, Sugars 15 g, Protein 3 g.

BUTTERMILK–ORANGE SCONES

Makes 9 servings • Serving size: 1 scone

Handle the dough as little as possible as you shape it to ensure that the scones bake up tender and flaky. Depending on what looks freshest in the market, you can use tangerines or clementines for the zest instead of oranges.

2 cups all-purpose flour

4 tablespoons granulated sugar, divided use

2 teaspoons baking powder

1/2 teaspoon baking soda

1/4 teaspoon salt

3 tablespoons 67% vegetable oil butter-flavored spread, chilled

2/3 cup low-fat buttermilk

1 large egg

1 teaspoon vanilla extract

1 tablespoon fresh grated orange zest

1. Preheat the oven to 375°F. Coat a baking sheet with cooking spray and set aside.

2. Combine the flour, 3 tablespoons of the sugar, baking powder, baking soda, salt, and butter-flavored spread in a food processor and pulse until spread is uniformly incorporated into the dry ingredients. Transfer the mixture to a large bowl and set aside.

3. Combine the buttermilk, egg, and vanilla in a small bowl and whisk to mix well. Stir in the orange zest. Add the buttermilk mixture to the flour mixture and stir just until moistened.

4. Transfer the dough to a lightly floured surface, sprinkle lightly with flour, and using floured hands, shape the dough into a 9-inch square. Cut the dough into 9 squares and transfer to the prepared pan, spacing about 1/2-inch apart. Sprinkle evenly with the remaining 1 tablespoon sugar. Bake 12 to 14 minutes, or until the tops of the scones are lightly browned. Serve immediately.

Exchanges: 2 Carbohydrate • 1/2 Fat
Calories 169, Calories from Fat 37, Total Fat 4 g, Saturated Fat 1 g, Cholesterol 24 mg, Sodium 273 mg, Total Carbohydrate 28 g, Dietary Fiber 1 g, Sugars 7 g, Protein 4 g.

DRIED APPLE–WALNUT SCONES

Makes 8 servings • Serving size: 1 scone

Make fast work of chopping dried apples by cutting them with kitchen shears instead of a knife. Enjoy these on a fall or winter day with a cup of hot tea or apple cider.

1/3 cup walnut pieces

1/4 cup unsweetened apple juice

1/4 cup dried apple slices, chopped

1 cup all-purpose flour

1/4 cup whole wheat flour

1/4 cup light brown sugar

1 teaspoon baking powder

1/4 teaspoon baking soda

1/4 teaspoon salt

1/4 teaspoon ground cinnamon

2 tablespoons 67% vegetable oil butter-flavored spread, chilled

1/3 cup low-fat buttermilk

1 large egg

1. Preheat the oven to 350°F. Place the nuts in a small baking pan. Bake, stirring once, 5 to 8 minutes or until nuts are lightly toasted. Set aside to cool. Finely chop cooled nuts. Increase the oven temperature to 375°F.

2. Place the apple juice in a small saucepan and heat over medium heat until hot, but not boiling. Remove from the heat and add the apples. Cover and let stand 10 minutes or until most of the juice is absorbed. Drain the apples and set aside.

3. Coat a baking pan with cooking spray and set aside.

4. Combine the all-purpose flour, whole wheat flour, brown sugar, baking powder, baking soda, salt, cinnamon, and butter-flavored spread in a food processor and pulse until the spread is uniformly incorporated into the dry ingredients. Transfer the mixture to a large bowl and set aside.

5. Combine the buttermilk and egg in a small bowl and whisk until well mixed. Add the buttermilk mixture, walnuts, and apples to the flour mixture and stir just until moistened.

6. Transfer the dough to a lightly floured surface, sprinkle lightly with flour, and using floured hands, shape the dough into an 8-inch circle. Cut into 8 wedges. Transfer the wedges to the prepared pan, spacing about 1/2 inch apart. Bake 12 to 14 minutes or until the tops of the scones are lightly browned. Serve immediately.

Exchanges: 1 1/2 Carbohydrate • 1 1/2 Fat
Calories 174, Calories from Fat 59, Total Fat 7 g, Saturated Fat 1 g, Cholesterol 27 mg, Sodium 206 mg, Total Carbohydrate 26 g, Dietary Fiber 2 g, Sugars 10 g, Protein 4 g.

Sweetie Pies

Apple Pie with Cinnamon Crunch Topping

Makes 8 servings • Serving size: 1 slice

Cereal adds a nice crunch to this simple, yet wonderful, pie. Don't worry about the seemingly large amount of apples used here—they'll cook down as the pie bakes.

Filling

6 medium Granny Smith apples (about 2 1/4 pounds), peeled, cored, and sliced into 1/4-inch-thick slices (about 7 cups)

2 teaspoons fresh grated lemon zest

1 tablespoon fresh lemon juice

1/2 cup granular no-calorie sweetener

2 tablespoons all-purpose flour

1/4 teaspoon salt

Cereal Topping

1/4 cup nut-like whole grain wheat and barley cereal

3 tablespoons light brown sugar

1/2 teaspoon ground cinnamon

1 1/2 tablespoons 67% vegetable oil butter-flavored spread, at room temperature

Crust

1 cup all-purpose flour

1/2 teaspoon salt

1/2 teaspoon baking powder

1/4 teaspoon baking soda

1/4 cup canola oil

3 tablespoons reduced-fat sour cream

Make Filling

1. Preheat the oven to 375°F.

2. Combine the apples, lemon zest, and lemon juice in a large bowl and toss to coat.

3. Combine the no-calorie sweetener, flour, and salt in a small bowl and whisk to mix well. Sprinkle over the apples and toss to coat. Set aside.

Make Topping

1. Combine the cereal, brown sugar, and cinnamon in a medium bowl and stir to mix well.

2. Add the butter-flavored spread and blend into dry ingredients using a pastry blender or your fingertips until the spread is uniformly incorporated. Set aside.

Make Crust

1. Coat a 9-inch glass pie plate with cooking spray and set aside.

2. Combine the flour, salt, baking powder, and baking soda in a medium bowl. Combine the oil and sour cream in a small bowl and whisk until well mixed. Add the oil mixture to the flour mixture and stir until a stiff dough forms. Shape the dough into a disk and place between 2 sheets of waxed paper.

3. Roll the dough to a 12-inch diameter circle. Remove the top layer of waxed paper and place the dough, with waxed paper facing up, into the prepared pie plate. Starting from the edge of the dough, gently remove the waxed paper. Fit the dough into the prepared pie plate, folding the edges under. Place the apple mixture in the crust. Sprinkle the topping over the apples.

4. Bake 30 to 35 minutes or until the crust is well browned. Remove the pie from the oven and cover loosely with foil. Return to the oven and bake 10 to 15 minutes longer or until the apples are tender. Cool completely on a wire rack.

Exchanges: 2 1/2 Carbohydrate • 1 1/2 Fat
Calories 248, Calories from Fat 87, Total Fat 10 g, Saturated Fat 1 g, Cholesterol 2 mg, Sodium 323 mg, Total Carbohydrate 40 g, Dietary Fiber 3 g, Sugars 21 g, Protein 3 g.

CHERRY AND TOASTED ALMOND PIE

Makes 8 servings • Serving size: 1 slice

This delicious pie makes the effort of pitting fresh cherries worth it.
Tie on an apron to protect your clothing from the juices and prepare for a treat!

Filling

1/2 cup granular no-calorie sweetener

1/4 cup cornstarch

Pinch of salt

2 pounds (about 6 cups) fresh sweet cherries, pitted or 6 cups unsweetened frozen cherries, thawed

1/2 teaspoon almond extract

Crust

1 cup all-purpose flour

1/2 teaspoon salt

1/2 teaspoon baking powder

1/4 teaspoon baking soda

1/4 cup canola oil

3 tablespoons reduced-fat sour cream

Topping

2 tablespoons slivered almonds

Make Filling

1. Preheat the oven to 400°F.

2. Combine the no-calorie sweetener, cornstarch, and salt in a large bowl and stir to mix well. Add the cherries and toss to coat. Sprinkle the cherry mixture with the extract and toss to coat. Set aside.

Make Crust

1. Coat a 9-inch glass pie plate with cooking spray and set aside.

2. Combine the flour, salt, baking powder, and baking soda in a medium bowl. Combine the oil and sour cream in a small bowl and whisk until well mixed. Add the oil mixture to the flour mixture and stir until a stiff dough forms. Shape the dough into a disk and place between 2 sheets of waxed paper.

3. Roll the dough to a 12-inch diameter circle. Remove the top layer of waxed paper and place the dough, with waxed paper facing up, into the prepared pie plate. Starting from the edge of the dough, gently remove the waxed paper. Fit the dough into the prepared pie plate, folding the edges under.

4. Spoon the cherry mixture into crust and bake 20 minutes. Remove the pie from the oven and reduce the oven temperature to 350°F. Cover pie loosely with foil and immediately return to the oven. Bake 25 to 30 minutes longer or until the fruit is bubbly. Maintain oven temperature.

Make Topping

1. Place the almonds in a small baking pan and bake at 350°F until lightly toasted, 6 to 8 minutes. Set the almonds aside to cool.

2. Cool the pie 1 hour on a wire rack before slicing. Sprinkle with almonds just before serving. Serve slightly warm or at room temperature.

Exchanges: 2 1/2 Carbohydrate • 1 1/2 Fat
Calories 232, Calories from Fat 85, Total Fat 9 g, Saturated Fat 1 g, Cholesterol 2 mg, Sodium 231 mg, Total Carbohydrate 35 g, Dietary Fiber 3 g, Sugars 17 g, Protein 4 g.

FRESH CRANBERRY–WALNUT PIE WITH SOUR CREAM TOPPING

Makes 8 servings • Serving size: 1 slice with 2 tablespoons topping

The cranberry filling of this pie is tart on its own, but paired with the maple syrup-sweetened crust and the sour cream topping, it's perfect. The topping is a wonderful faux whipped cream; use it to accompany fresh fruit, garnish pies or brownies, or dress up a slice of plain cake. It's quick and easy to prepare, but lasts only a couple of hours in the refrigerator, so don't make it too far in advance.

Crust

9 low-fat graham crackers, crumbled (use 9 whole rectangles)

1/4 cup maple syrup

Filling

4 cups fresh cranberries, divided use

1/2 cup granular no-calorie sweetener

1/4 cup light brown sugar

1/4 cup maple syrup

Pinch of salt

2 teaspoons fresh grated orange zest

1/2 cup chopped walnuts

1 teaspoon vanilla extract

Topping

1/4 cup reduced-fat sour cream

2 tablespoons granular no-calorie sweetener

1/2 teaspoon vanilla extract

2 tablespoons cold water

1/2 tablespoon 100% dried egg whites or meringue powder

2 tablespoons granulated sugar

Make Crust

1. Preheat the oven to 350°F. Coat a 9-inch glass pie plate with cooking spray and set aside.

2. Place crumbled graham crackers in a food processor and process until finely ground. Transfer to a medium bowl and stir in maple syrup. Coat your hands lightly with cooking spray and press the mixture into the bottom and up the sides of the prepared pie plate.

3. Bake 10 to 12 minutes or until the crust is lightly browned. Cool completely on a wire rack.

Make Filling

1. Combine 3 cups of the cranberries, the no-calorie sweetener, brown sugar, maple syrup, and salt in a medium saucepan and cook over medium heat, stirring often, 8 to 10 minutes or until the cranberries pop. Remove from the heat and stir in the orange zest. Transfer to a medium bowl and cool completely.

2. Place the remaining 1 cup cranberries in a food processor and pulse until coarsely chopped. Stir the cranberries, walnuts, and vanilla into the cooled filling mixture.

3. Spoon into the prepared crust, cover, and refrigerate 4 hours or overnight. Serve each slice with 2 tablespoons topping.

Make Topping

1. Combine the sour cream, no-calorie sweetener, and vanilla in a medium bowl and stir to mix well. Set aside.

2. Combine the water and dried egg whites in a medium bowl and beat at high speed for 5 minutes or until foamy. Gradually beat in the sugar, beating 5 minutes longer or until stiff, glossy, and bright white.

3. Gently fold the meringue mixture into the sour cream mixture in four additions, mixing well after each addition. Cover and refrigerate up to 2 hours.

Exchanges: 3 Carbohydrate • 1 Fat
Calories 253, Calories from Fat 61, Total Fat 7 g, Saturated Fat 1 g, Cholesterol 3 mg, Sodium 141 mg, Total Carbohydrate 47 g, Dietary Fiber 3 g, Sugars 33 g, Protein 3 g.

Lemon–Lime Meringue Pie

Makes 8 servings • Serving size: 1 slice

A crown of airy meringue tops off a tangy citrus filling that's as good as the classic, yet high-fat, version of lemon meringue pie. Don't be concerned about the thin consistency of the filling; it thickens and slices perfectly after chilling.

Crust

1 cup all-purpose flour

1/2 teaspoon salt

1/2 teaspoon baking powder

1/4 teaspoon baking soda

1/4 cup canola oil

3 tablespoons reduced-fat sour cream

Filling

1/2 cup granulated sugar

1/2 cup granular no-calorie sweetener

1/4 cup cornstarch

1 3/4 cups water

2 egg yolks

1/3 cup fresh lemon juice

1/3 cup fresh lime juice

2 teaspoons fresh grated lemon zest

2 teaspoons fresh grated lime zest

Meringue

4 egg whites

1/2 teaspoon cream of tartar

1/2 teaspoon vanilla extract

1/4 cup granulated sugar

Make Crust

1. Preheat the oven to 375°F. Coat a 9-inch glass pie plate with cooking spray and set aside.

2. Combine the flour, salt, baking powder, and baking soda in a medium bowl. Combine the oil and sour cream in a small bowl and whisk until well mixed. Add the oil mixture to the flour mixture and stir until a stiff dough forms. Shape dough into a disk and place between 2 sheets of waxed paper.

3. Roll dough to a 12-inch diameter circle. Remove the top layer of waxed paper and place the dough, with waxed paper facing up, into the prepared pie plate. Starting from the edge of the dough, gently remove the waxed paper. Fit the dough into the prepared pie plate, folding the edges under. Prick the bottom all over with a fork. Bake 10 to 12 minutes or until the crust is lightly browned. Reduce the oven temperature to 350°F.

Make Filling

1. Combine the sugar, no-calorie sweetener, cornstarch, water, and egg yolks in a medium heavy-bottomed saucepan and whisk until the cornstarch dissolves.

2. Cook over medium heat, whisking constantly, about 6 minutes or until the mixture comes to a boil and thickens. Remove the filling from the heat and stir in the lemon juice, lime juice, lemon zest, and lime zest. Pour into the hot crust.

Make Meringue

1. Combine the egg whites and cream of tartar in a large bowl and beat at high speed until foamy. Beat in the vanilla. Gradually add the sugar and beat at high speed until stiff peaks form.

2. Carefully spread the meringue evenly over the hot filling, mounding in the center and spreading to the edges of the filling. Bake 15 minutes. Cool completely on a wire rack. Loosely cover and refrigerate 4 hours or until firm.

Exchanges: 2 1/2 Carbohydrate • 1 1/2 Fat
Calories 245, Calories from Fat 79, Total Fat 9 g, Saturated Fat 1 g, Cholesterol 55 mg, Sodium 244 mg, Total Carbohydrate 37 g, Dietary Fiber 1 g, Sugars 21 g, Protein 4 g.

Banana Meringue Pie

Makes: 8 servings • Serving size: 1 slice

Fat-free meringue stands in for the more typical (and high-fat) whipped cream topping
on a classic banana cream pie. This version is just as good, but with much less fat.
Make the crust and the filling a day ahead, but top the pie with meringue
no more than a couple of hours before serving.

Crust

9 low-fat graham crackers, crumbled
(use 9 whole rectangles)

2 tablespoons 67% vegetable oil butter-
flavored spread, melted and cooled

1 egg white

Filling

3 cups fat-free milk

1 large egg

1/2 cup granular no-calorie sweetener

1/3 cup cornstarch

1/4 cup granulated sugar

Pinch of salt

2 teaspoons vanilla extract

1 1/2 cups sliced bananas

Meringue

1/4 cup cold water

1 tablespoon 100% dried egg whites or
meringue powder

1/2 teaspoon vanilla extract

2 tablespoons granulated sugar

Make Crust

1. Preheat the oven to 350°F. Coat a 9-inch glass pie plate with cooking spray and set aside.

2. Place crumbled graham crackers in a food processor and process until finely ground. Transfer to a medium bowl and stir in butter-flavored spread and egg white. Coat your hands lightly with cooking spray and press mixture into the bottom and up the sides of the prepared pie plate.

3. Bake 8 to 10 minutes or until the crust is lightly browned (small cracks may appear). Cool completely on a wire rack.

Make Filling

1. Combine the milk, egg, no-calorie sweetener, cornstarch, sugar, and salt in a medium heavy-bottomed saucepan and whisk until the cornstarch dissolves. Cook over medium heat, whisking constantly, about 6 minutes or until the mixture comes to a boil and thickens.

2. Transfer to a medium bowl and cover the surface of the filling with plastic wrap to prevent a skin from forming. Cool to room temperature and stir in the vanilla. Stir in the bananas and spoon the filling into the prepared crust. Cover the surface of the filling with plastic wrap and refrigerate 4 hours or until firm.

Make Meringue

1. Preheat the broiler.

2. Combine the water and dried egg whites in a large bowl and beat at high speed for 5 minutes or until foamy. Beat in the vanilla. Gradually beat in the sugar, beating 5 minutes longer or until stiff, glossy, and bright white.

3. Top the pie with the meringue, mounding in the center and spreading to the edges of the filling. Broil 1 to 2 minutes or until the meringue is lightly browned.

Exchanges: 2 1/2 Carbohydrate • 1 Fat
Calories 225, Calories from Fat 35, Total Fat 4 g, Saturated Fat 1 g, Cholesterol 30 mg, Sodium 200 mg, Total Carbohydrate 42 g, Dietary Fiber 1 g, Sugars 24 g, Protein 7 g.

PEACHES AND CREAM PIE

Makes 8 servings • Serving size: 1 slice

Tart–sweet peaches make a delightful contrast to a rich sour cream filling in
this summer pie. With less fat and carbohydrate than other versions,
you can afford to enjoy it throughout peach season.

Crust

9 low-fat graham crackers, crumbled
(use 9 whole rectangles)

1/2 teaspoon ground nutmeg

2 tablespoons 67% vegetable oil butter-
flavored spread, melted and cooled

1 egg white

Filling

2 cups fat-free milk

1 egg yolk

2/3 cup granular no-calorie sweetener

1/4 cup granulated sugar

1/4 cup cornstarch

Pinch of salt

3 tablespoons reduced-fat sour cream

1 teaspoon vanilla extract

Topping

3 medium ripe but firm peaches
(about 1 pound), peeled and thinly sliced

Make Crust

1. Preheat the oven to 350°F. Coat a 9-inch glass pie plate with cooking spray and set aside.

2. Place the crumbled graham crackers and nutmeg in a food processor and process until finely ground. Transfer to a medium bowl and stir in the butter-flavored spread and egg white. Coat your hands lightly with cooking spray and press the mixture into the bottom and up the sides of the prepared pie plate.

3. Bake 10 to 12 minutes or until the crust is lightly browned (small cracks may appear). Cool completely on a wire rack.

Make Filling

1. Combine the milk, egg yolk, no-calorie sweetener, sugar, cornstarch, and salt in a medium heavy-bottomed saucepan and whisk until the cornstarch dissolves. Cook over medium heat, whisking constantly, about 6 minutes or until the mixture comes to a boil and thickens.

2. Remove from the heat and whisk in the sour cream. Transfer to a medium bowl and cover the surface of the pudding with plastic wrap to prevent a skin from forming. Cool to room temperature and stir in the vanilla. Spoon into the prepared crust. Cover and refrigerate 2 hours or until firm. Top with peach slices just before serving.

Exchanges: 2 1/2 Carbohydrate • 1/2 Fat
Calories 200, Calories from Fat 45, Total Fat 5 g, Saturated Fat 1 g, Cholesterol 30 mg, Sodium 193 mg, Total Carbohydrate 35 g, Dietary Fiber 1 g, Sugars 20 g, Protein 5 g.

CHOCOLATE GRAHAM PIE

Makes 8 servings • Serving size: 1 slice

A graham cracker crust and a custardy chocolate filling team up to make
this an old-fashioned treat.

Crust

9 low-fat graham crackers, crumbled
(use 9 whole rectangles)

2 tablespoons 67% vegetable oil butter-
flavored spread, melted and cooled

1 egg white

Filling

3 cups fat-free milk

1/2 cup fat-free sweetened condensed milk

1 large egg

1/2 cup granular no-calorie sweetener

1/2 cup unsweetened cocoa

1/3 cup cornstarch

Pinch of salt

2 teaspoons vanilla extract

Garnish

Semisweet chocolate shavings (optional)

Make Crust

1. Preheat the oven to 350°F. Coat a 9-inch glass pie plate with cooking spray and set aside.

2. Place crumbled graham crackers in a food processor and process until finely ground. Transfer to a medium bowl and stir in butter-flavored spread and egg white. Coat your hands lightly with cooking spray and press the mixture into the bottom and up the sides of the prepared pie plate.

3. Bake 8 to 10 minutes or until the crust is lightly browned (small cracks may appear). Cool completely on a wire rack.

Make Filling

1. Combine the fat-free milk, condensed milk, egg, no-calorie sweetener, cocoa, cornstarch, and salt in a medium heavy-bottomed saucepan and whisk until the cornstarch dissolves. Cook over medium heat, whisking constantly, about 6 minutes or until the mixture comes to a boil and thickens.

2. Transfer to a medium bowl and cover the surface of the filling with plastic wrap to prevent a skin from forming. Cool to room temperature and stir in the vanilla. Spoon into the crust, cover, and refrigerate 2 hours or until firm. Garnish with semi-sweet chocolate shavings, if desired.

Exchanges: 2 1/2 Carbohydrate • 1 Fat
Calories 225, Calories from Fat 40, Total Fat 5 g, Saturated Fat 1 g, Cholesterol 30 mg, Sodium 233 mg, Total Carbohydrate 39 g, Dietary Fiber 2 g, Sugars 23 g, Protein 8 g.

Sweet Potato Praline Pie

Makes 8 servings • Serving size: 1 slice

A crunchy pecan praline topping sets off a silky sweet potato filling in this homey Southern-style pie. It's a welcome slice of sweet comfort to serve throughout the fall and winter.

Filling

2 large sweet potatoes (about 1 1/4 pounds)

1/2 cup fat-free milk

1/4 cup granular no-calorie sweetener

1/4 cup light brown sugar

1 large egg

1 egg white

1 teaspoon vanilla extract

1 teaspoon ground cinnamon

1/2 teaspoon ground nutmeg

1/2 teaspoon ground ginger

Pinch of salt

Crust

1 cup all-purpose flour

1/2 teaspoon salt

1/2 teaspoon baking powder

1/4 teaspoon baking soda

1/4 cup canola oil

3 tablespoons reduced-fat sour cream

Praline

2 tablespoons granulated sugar

1/4 cup chopped pecans

Make Filling

1. Pierce the potatoes several times with a fork. Microwave on high 8 minutes per side or until tender. Cut open and cool completely. Spoon the potato flesh into a bowl and mash until smooth. Measure enough potato puree to equal 1 1/2 cups.

2. Combine 1 1/2 cups potato puree and the milk in a food processor and process until the mixture is smooth. Transfer to a medium bowl and stir in the no-calorie sweetener, brown sugar, egg, egg white, vanilla, cinnamon, nutmeg, ginger, and salt. Set aside.

Make Crust

1. Preheat the oven to 350°F.

2. Coat a 9-inch glass pie plate with cooking spray and set aside.

3. Combine the flour, salt, baking powder, and baking soda in a medium bowl. Combine the oil and sour cream in a small bowl and whisk until smooth. Add the oil mixture to the flour mixture and stir until a stiff dough forms. Shape the dough into a disk and place between 2 sheets of waxed paper.

4. Roll dough to a 12-inch diameter circle. Remove the top layer of waxed paper and place the dough, with waxed paper facing up, into the prepared pie plate. Starting from the edge of the dough, gently remove the waxed paper. Fit the dough into the prepared pie plate, folding the edges under. Pour the filling into the prepared crust. Bake 30 minutes or until the crust is browned and the filling is set. Cool the pie completely on a wire rack.

Make Praline

1. Place a sheet of parchment paper on a heat-proof surface.

2. Cook the sugar in a medium heavy-bottomed skillet over medium-high heat 3 minutes or until the sugar melts. Remove from the heat and quickly stir in the pecans. Immediately spoon the mixture onto parchment paper and cool completely. Break into small pieces before sprinkling on the pie just before serving.

Exchanges: 2 1/2 Carbohydrate • 2 Fat
Calories 275, Calories from Fat 98, Total Fat 11 g, Saturated Fat 1 g, Cholesterol 29 mg, Sodium 265 mg, Total Carbohydrate 40 g, Dietary Fiber 2 g, Sugars 16 g, Protein 5 g.

CREAMY STRAWBERRY PIE

Makes 8 servings • Serving size: 1 slice

With frozen strawberries, you can enjoy this mile-high pie year round.
If it's springtime, though, be sure to adorn each serving with tumble of sliced fresh berries.

Crust

1 cup all-purpose flour

1/2 teaspoon salt

1/2 teaspoon baking powder

1/4 teaspoon baking soda

1/4 cup canola oil

3 tablespoons reduced-fat sour cream

Filling

1 (16-ounce) package frozen unsweetened strawberries, thawed

1/2 cup 1% low-fat milk

1 envelope unflavored gelatin

1/2 cup granular no-calorie sweetener

1/3 cup fat-free sweetened condensed milk

1/4 cup cold water

1 tablespoon 100% dried egg whites or meringue powder

1/2 teaspoon vanilla extract

2 tablespoons granulated sugar

Garnish

Fresh sliced strawberries (optional)

Make Crust

1. Preheat the oven to 375°F. Coat a 9-inch glass pie plate with cooking spray and set aside.

2. Combine the flour, salt, baking powder, and baking soda in a medium bowl. Combine the oil and sour cream in a small bowl and whisk until smooth. Add the oil mixture to the flour mixture and stir until a stiff dough forms. Shape the dough into a disk and place between 2 sheets of waxed paper.

3. Roll the dough to a 12-inch diameter circle. Remove the top layer of waxed paper and place the dough, with waxed paper facing up, into the prepared pie plate. Starting from the edge of the dough, gently remove the waxed paper. Fit the dough into the prepared pie plate, folding the edges under. Prick the bottom all over with a fork. Bake 10 to 12 minutes or until the crust is lightly browned. Cool completely on a wire rack.

Make Filling

1. Place the strawberries in a food processor and process until smooth. Set aside.

2. Pour the milk into a medium saucepan. Sprinkle the gelatin over the milk and let stand 2 minutes to soften. Cook the mixture over medium heat, stirring often, about 2 minutes or until the gelatin dissolves. Remove from the heat and pour into a large bowl. Stir in the strawberry puree, no-calorie sweetener, and sweetened condensed milk. Set aside.

3. Combine the water and dried egg whites in a large bowl and beat at high speed for 5 minutes or until foamy. Beat in vanilla. Gradually beat in sugar, beating 5 minutes longer or until stiff, glossy, and bright white. Gently fold the meringue into the strawberry mixture in four additions, mixing until no white streaks remain.

4. Refrigerate the filling, stirring occasionally, 1 1/2 hours or until the filling begins to thicken. Spoon the filling into the prepared crust, mounding in the center. Cover the surface of the pie with plastic wrap and refrigerate 4 hours or until firm. Garnish with fresh sliced strawberries, if desired.

Exchanges: 2 Carbohydrate • 1 1/2 Fat
Calories 210, Calories from Fat 69, Total Fat 8 g, Saturated Fat 1 g, Cholesterol 3 mg, Sodium 246 mg, Total Carbohydrate 31 g, Dietary Fiber 2 g, Sugars 16 g, Protein 5 g.

Tropical Cloud Pie

Makes 8 servings • Serving size: 1 slice

Like a piña colada in a crust, this refreshing pie is the perfect ending for a Tex-Mex meal.

Crust

9 low-fat graham crackers, crumbled
(use 9 whole rectangles)

1/2 teaspoon ground nutmeg

2 tablespoons 67% vegetable oil butter-
flavored spread, melted and cooled

1 egg white

Filling

1/2 cup frozen pineapple juice
concentrate, thawed

1 envelope unflavored gelatin

1/2 cup granular no-calorie sweetener

1/4 cup granulated sugar

Pinch of salt

1 1/2 cups fat-free milk

1/4 cup reduced-fat sour cream

1/2 cup refrigerated liquid egg whites

Garnish

1 tablespoon sweetened flaked coconut,
toasted

Make Crust

1. Preheat the oven to 350°F. Coat a 9-inch glass pie plate with cooking spray and set aside.

2. Place the crumbled graham crackers and nutmeg in a food processor and process until finely ground. Transfer to a medium bowl and stir in the butter-flavored spread and egg white. Coat your hands lightly with cooking spray and press the mixture into the bottom and up the sides of the prepared pie plate.

3. Bake 10 to 12 minutes or until the crust is lightly browned (small cracks may appear). Cool completely on a wire rack.

Make Filling

1. Pour the pineapple juice concentrate into a medium saucepan. Sprinkle the gelatin over the juice and let stand 2 minutes to soften. Add the no calorie-sweetener, sugar, and salt and cook the mixture over medium heat, stirring often, about 2 minutes or until the sugar dissolves. Remove from the heat and pour into a large bowl. Whisk in the milk and sour cream.

2. Place the egg whites in a large bowl and beat at high speed 2 to 3 minutes or until the whites have doubled in volume and soft peaks form. Gently fold the egg whites into the milk mixture in four additions, mixing until no white streaks remain.

3. Refrigerate the filling, stirring occasionally, 1 1/2 hours or until the filling begins to thicken. Spoon the filling into the prepared crust. Cover the surface of the pie with plastic wrap and refrigerate 4 hours or until firm. Sprinkle with toasted coconut just before serving.

Exchanges: 2 Carbohydrate • 1 Fat
Calories 195, Calories from Fat 39, Total Fat 4 g, Saturated Fat 1 g, Cholesterol 4 mg, Sodium 218 mg, Total Carbohydrate 33 g, Dietary Fiber 1 g, Sugars 22 g, Protein 6 g.

Pumpkin Chiffon Pie

Makes 8 servings • Serving size: 1 slice

Carb and calorie counters won't feel deprived when you serve slices of this creamy, subtly spiced pie at your holiday dinner. It's perfect for entertaining because it's completely make-ahead and guaranteed to win compliments for the cook.

Crust

9 low-fat graham crackers, crumbled (use 9 whole rectangles)

2 tablespoons 67% vegetable oil butter-flavored spread, melted and cooled

1 egg white

Filling

1/2 cup 1% low-fat milk

1 envelope unflavored gelatin

1/2 cup light brown sugar, divided use

1/4 cup granular no-calorie sweetener

3/4 teaspoon ground cinnamon

1/2 teaspoon ground ginger

1/4 teaspoon ground nutmeg

1/4 teaspoon salt

1 (15-ounce) can 100% pure pumpkin (not pumpkin pie filling)

1/4 cup cold water

1 tablespoon 100% dried egg whites or meringue powder

Make Crust

1. Preheat the oven to 350°F. Coat a 9-inch glass pie plate with cooking spray and set aside.

2. Place the crumbled graham crackers in a food processor and process until finely ground. Transfer to a medium bowl and stir in the butter-flavored spread and egg white. Coat your hands lightly with cooking spray and press the mixture into the bottom and up the sides of the prepared pie plate.

3. Bake 8 to 10 minutes or until the crust is lightly browned (small cracks may appear). Cool completely on a wire rack.

Make Filling

1. Pour the milk into a medium saucepan, sprinkle with the gelatin, and let stand 2 minutes to soften. Add 1/4 cup of the brown sugar, the no calorie-sweetener, cinnamon, ginger, nutmeg, and salt and cook the mixture over medium heat, stirring often, about 2 minutes or until the sugar dissolves. Remove from the heat and pour the mixture into a large bowl. Whisk in the pumpkin.

2. Combine the water and dried egg whites in a large bowl and beat at high speed for 5 minutes or until foamy. Gradually beat in the sugar, beating 5 minutes longer or until stiff, glossy, and bright white. Gently fold the meringue mixture into the pumpkin mixture in four additions.

3. Refrigerate the filling, stirring occasionally, 1 1/2 hours or until the filling begins to thicken. Spoon the filling into the prepared crust. Cover the surface of the pie with plastic wrap and refrigerate 4 hours or until firm.

Exchanges: 2 Carbohydrate• 1/2 Fat
Calories 168, Calories from Fat 25, Total Fat 3 g, Saturated Fat 1 g, Cholesterol 1 mg, Sodium 236 mg, Total Carbohydrate 34 g, Dietary Fiber 2 g, Sugars 21 g, Protein 4 g.

Rustic Plum Crostata

Makes 6 servings • Serving size: 1 slice

Think of a crostata as a laid-back pie. Of Italian heritage, it is customarily baked free-form on a baking sheet instead of in a pie plate. So, don't fuss over making the crust look perfect—the imperfections only add to its charm. If ripe plums are not available at the market, buy them a couple of days in advance and store at room temperature until the flesh gives slightly to gentle pressure.

Filling

1 pound ripe plums, pitted and sliced (about 2 3/4 cups)

1 teaspoon fresh grated lemon zest

3 tablespoons granulated sugar, divided use

1 tablespoon all-purpose flour

1/4 teaspoon ground nutmeg

Crust

1 cup all-purpose flour

1/2 teaspoon salt

1/2 teaspoon baking powder

1/4 teaspoon baking soda

1/4 cup canola oil

3 tablespoons reduced-fat sour cream

1 egg white, beaten

Make Filling

1. Preheat the oven to 400°F.

2. Place the plums and lemon zest in a large bowl and toss to combine.

3. Combine 2 1/2 tablespoons of the sugar, the flour, and nutmeg in a small bowl and stir to mix well. Sprinkle over the plum mixture and toss to coat. Set aside.

Make Crust

1. Line a baking pan with parchment paper and set aside.

2. Combine the flour, salt, baking powder, and baking soda in a medium bowl. Combine the oil and sour cream in a small bowl and whisk until well mixed. Add the oil mixture to the flour mixture and stir until a stiff dough forms. Shape the dough into a disk and place between 2 sheets of waxed paper.

3. Roll the dough to a 12-inch diameter circle. Remove the top layer of waxed paper and place the dough, with waxed paper facing up, into the parchment-lined pan. Starting from the edge of the dough, gently remove the waxed paper.

4. Place the filling in a mound in the center of the crust. Using the parchment paper to lift the crust, carefully fold the crust over the edge of the filling. Brush the crust with egg white and sprinkle with the remaining 1/2 tablespoon of sugar.

5. Bake for 25 to 30 minutes or until the crust is lightly browned and the fruit is bubbly. Cool in the pan on a wire rack. Serve warm or at room temperature.

Exchanges: 2 Carbohydrate • 2 Fat
Calories 232, Calories from Fat 91, Total Fat 10 g, Saturated Fat 1 g, Cholesterol 3 mg, Sodium 292 mg, Total Carbohydrate 32 g, Dietary Fiber 2 g, Sugars 14 g, Protein 4 g.

Sugar-and-Spice Pear Crostata

Makes 6 servings • Serving size: 1 slice

This quick and easy pleated-edged pie is good anytime you need a
delicious, informal fall dessert.

Filling

2 tablespoons granulated sugar, divided use

1 tablespoon all-purpose flour

1/4 teaspoon ground cinnamon

2 large ripe but firm pears (about 1 pound),
peeled and sliced (about 2 1/2 cups)

Crust

1 cup all-purpose flour

1/2 teaspoon salt

1/2 teaspoon baking powder

1/4 teaspoon baking soda

1/4 cup canola oil

3 tablespoons reduced-fat sour cream

1 egg white, lightly beaten

Make Filling

1. Preheat the oven to 400°F.

2. Combine 1 1/2 tablespoons of the sugar, the flour, and cinnamon in a large bowl and stir to mix well. Add the pears and toss to coat. Set aside.

Make Crust

1. Line a baking pan with parchment paper and set aside.

2. Combine the flour, salt, baking powder, and baking soda in a medium bowl. Combine the oil and sour cream in a small bowl and whisk until well mixed. Add the oil mixture to the flour mixture and stir until a stiff dough forms. Shape the dough into a disk and place between 2 sheets of waxed paper.

3. Roll the dough to a 12-inch diameter circle. Remove the top layer of waxed paper and place the dough, with waxed paper facing up, into the parchment-lined pan. Starting from the edge of the dough, gently remove the waxed paper.

4. Place the filling in a mound in the center of the crust. Using the parchment paper to lift the crust, carefully fold the crust over the edge of the filling. Brush the crust with egg white and sprinkle with the remaining 1/2 tablespoon of sugar.

5. Bake for 25 to 30 minutes or until the crust is lightly browned and the fruit is bubbly. Cool in the pan on a wire rack. Serve warm or at room temperature.

Exchanges: 2 Carbohydrate • 2 Fat
Calories 231, Calories from Fat 90, Total Fat 10 g, Saturated Fat 1 g, Cholesterol 3 mg, Sodium 293 mg, Total Carbohydrate 33 g, Dietary Fiber 3 g, Sugars 12 g, Protein 4 g.

Fruit Orchard Pot Pies

Makes 8 servings • Serving size: 1 pot pie

When rustling fall leaves bring on a craving for the fruits of the season's harvest, make these juicy bowls of goodness. You can use all apples or all pears if you wish, and dried cranberries or raisins can stand in for the dried cherries.

Filling

2 tablespoons light brown sugar

1 tablespoon all-purpose flour

1/4 teaspoon ground nutmeg

2 medium ripe but firm pears, peeled and chopped

2 medium Granny Smith apples, peeled and chopped

1/4 cup dried cherries

8 tablespoons unsweetened apple juice, divided use

Topping

3/4 cup all-purpose flour

2 tablespoons granulated sugar

2 tablespoons granular no-calorie sweetener

1 teaspoon baking powder

1/2 teaspoon baking soda

1/4 teaspoon salt

2 tablespoons 67% vegetable oil butter-flavored spread, chilled

1/4 cup low-fat buttermilk

Make Filling

1. Preheat the oven to 350°F. Coat 8 (1-cup) custard cups or ovenproof bowls with cooking spray and set aside.

2. Combine brown sugar, flour, and nutmeg in a large bowl and stir to mix well. Add pears, apples, and cherries and toss to coat. Spoon about 1/2 cup of fruit mixture into each of the prepared custard cups. Drizzle each one with 1 tablespoon of the apple juice.

Make Topping

1. Combine the flour, sugar, no-calorie sweetener, baking powder, baking soda, and salt in a large bowl. Add the butter-flavored spread and blend into dry ingredients using a pastry blender or your fingertips until the spread is uniformly incorporated. Add the buttermilk and stir just until moistened. Drop the batter evenly onto the fruit mixture.

2. Place the custard cups on a baking sheet and bake for 25 to 30 minutes or until the topping is well-browned and the fruit is tender. Serve warm.

Exchanges: 2 Carbohydrate • 1/2 Fat
Calories 159, Calories from Fat 24, Total Fat 3 g, Saturated Fat 1 g, Cholesterol 0 mg, Sodium 231 mg, Total Carbohydrate 33 g, Dietary Fiber 2 g, Sugars 19 g, Protein 2 g.

COCONUT CREAM PIE

Makes 8 servings • Serving size: 1 slice

Sheets of phyllo dough make a lacy-looking (and low-fat!) crust for a
rich-tasting coconut custard filling.

Crust

4 frozen phyllo sheets, thawed
(14 × 18 inches each)

Filling

1 1/2 cups fat-free milk

1/2 cup light coconut milk

1 egg yolk

2/3 cup granular
no-calorie sweetener

1/4 cup granulated sugar

1/4 cup cornstarch

Pinch of salt

1 teaspoon coconut extract

Garnish

1 tablespoon sweetened
flaked coconut, toasted

Make Crust

1. Preheat the oven to 375°F. Coat a 9-inch glass pie plate
   with cooking spray.

2. Place one sheet of phyllo in the pie plate and lightly coat with
   cooking spray. Repeat with the remaining sheets, coating each
   layer with cooking spray, and placing the sheets at an angle
   across each other. Gently ruffle the overhanging edges of the
   phyllo onto the rim of the pie plate. Prick the bottom of the
   crust all over with a fork. Bake 8 to 10 minutes or until the
   crust is lightly browned. Cool in the pan on a wire rack.

Make Filling

1. Combine the milk, coconut milk, egg yolk, no-calorie sweetener, sugar, cornstarch, and salt in a medium heavy-bottomed
   saucepan and whisk until the cornstarch dissolves. Cook over
   medium heat, whisking constantly, about 6 minutes or until
   the mixture comes to a boil and thickens.

2. Transfer to a medium bowl and cover the surface of the
   filling with plastic wrap to prevent a skin from forming.
   Cool to room temperature, stir in the coconut extract,
   and spoon into the prepared crust. Cover and refrigerate
   2 hours. Top with toasted coconut just before serving.

Exchanges: 1 1/2 Carbohydrate
Calories 120, Calories from Fat 16, Total Fat 2 g, Saturated Fat 1 g, Cholesterol 27 mg,
Sodium 111 mg, Total Carbohydrate 22 g, Dietary Fiber 0 g, Sugars 11 g, Protein 3 g.

Smart Tarts

Fudgy Chocolate Tart

Makes 10 servings • Serving size: 1 slice

For company, shower this tart with curls of dark and white chocolate for a stunning presentation. It's bursting with chocolate flavor, so your family won't mind having it plain!

Crust

1 cup all-purpose flour

1/2 teaspoon salt

1/2 teaspoon baking powder

1/4 teaspoon baking soda

1/4 cup canola oil

3 tablespoons reduced-fat sour cream

Filling

2 cups fat-free milk

1 large egg

2/3 cup granular no-calorie sweetener

1/3 cup unsweetened cocoa

1/4 cup granulated sugar

1/4 cup cornstarch

Pinch of salt

2 teaspoons vanilla extract

Make Crust

1. Preheat the oven to 400°F. Coat a 9-inch tart pan with removable bottom with cooking spray and set aside.

2. Combine the flour, salt, baking powder, and baking soda in a medium bowl and whisk to mix well. Combine the oil and sour cream in a small bowl and whisk until smooth. Add the oil mixture to the flour mixture and stir until a stiff dough forms. Shape the dough into a disk and place between 2 sheets of waxed paper.

3. Roll the dough to a 12-inch diameter circle. Remove the top layer of waxed paper and place the dough, with waxed paper facing up, into the prepared pan. Starting from the edge of the dough, gently remove the waxed paper. Trim the edges of the crust and prick the bottom all over with a fork. Bake 10 to 12 minutes or until the crust is lightly browned. Cool completely on a wire rack.

Make Filling

1. Combine the milk, egg, no-calorie sweetener, cocoa, sugar, cornstarch, and salt in a medium heavy-bottomed saucepan and whisk until the cornstarch dissolves. Cook over medium heat, whisking constantly, about 6 minutes or until the mixture comes to a boil and thickens.

2. Transfer to a medium bowl and cover the surface of the filling with plastic wrap to prevent a skin from forming. Cool to room temperature and stir in the vanilla. Spoon into the prepared crust, cover, and refrigerate 2 hours or until firm.

Exchanges: 1 1/2 Carbohydrate • 1 Fat
Calories 172, Calories from Fat 62, Total Fat 7 g, Saturated Fat 1 g, Cholesterol 24 mg, Sodium 219 mg, Total Carbohydrate 24 g, Dietary Fiber 1 g, Sugars 10 g, Protein 5 g.

Orange Blossom Tart

Makes 10 servings • Serving size: 1 slice

The contrast between the crisp crust, smooth filling, and juicy orange topping make this tart a textural delight. If navel oranges are not at their best in the market, you can make it in summer and fall with Valencia oranges.

Crust

9 low-fat graham crackers, crumbled (use 9 whole rectangles)

2 tablespoons 67% vegetable oil butter-flavored spread, melted and cooled

1 egg white

Filling

2 cups fresh-squeezed orange juice

1 large egg

1/4 cup granulated sugar

1/4 cup cornstarch

Pinch of salt

1 tablespoon fresh grated orange zest

Topping

2 large navel oranges

Make Crust

1. Preheat the oven to 350°F. Coat a 9-inch tart pan with removable bottom with cooking spray and set aside.

2. Place the crumbled graham crackers in a food processor and process until finely ground. Transfer to a medium bowl and stir in the butter-flavored spread and egg white. Coat your hands lightly with cooking spray and press the mixture into the bottom and up the sides of the prepared pan.

3. Place the tart pan on a baking sheet and bake 8 to 10 minutes or until the crust is lightly browned (small cracks may appear). Cool completely on a wire rack.

Make Filling

1. Combine the orange juice, egg, sugar, cornstarch, and salt in a medium heavy-bottomed saucepan and whisk until smooth. Cook over medium heat, whisking constantly, about 6 minutes or until the mixture comes to a boil and thickens.

2. Remove from the heat and stir in the orange zest. Transfer to a medium bowl and cover the surface of the filling with plastic wrap to prevent a skin from forming. Cool to room temperature. Spoon into the prepared crust, cover, and refrigerate 2 hours or until firm.

Make Topping

1. Cut a thin slice from the top and bottom of each of the oranges, exposing the flesh. Stand each fruit upright, and using a sharp knife, thickly cut off the peel, following the contour of the fruit and removing all the white pith and membrane. Holding the fruit over a bowl, carefully cut along both sides of each section to free it from the membrane. Discard any seeds and let the sections fall into the bowl.

2. Place the orange sections in a single layer on several thicknesses of paper towels. Gently blot with additional paper towels. Arrange the orange sections on the tart just before serving.

Exchanges: 2 Carbohydrate • 1 Fat
Calories 152, Calories from Fat 31, Total Fat 3 g, Saturated Fat 1 g, Cholesterol 21 mg, Sodium 132 mg, Total Carbohydrate 29 g, Dietary Fiber 1 g, Sugars 17 g, Protein 3 g.

Strawberry–Cream Cheese Tart

Makes 10 servings • Serving size: 1 slice

A small amount of strawberry preserves in the filling give this tart a blush of color
and a punch of berry flavor. Serve it in winter minus the fresh strawberries,
but with a drizzle of sugar-free chocolate syrup instead.

Crust

9 low-fat graham crackers, crumbled
(use 9 whole rectangles)

2 tablespoons 67% vegetable oil butter-
flavored spread, melted and cooled

1 egg white

Filling

2 cups fat-free milk

1 egg yolk

1/3 cup granular no-calorie sweetener

1/4 cup granulated sugar

1/4 cup cornstarch

Pinch of salt

1/4 cup reduced-sugar strawberry preserves

3 tablespoons reduced-fat cream cheese

1 teaspoon vanilla extract

Topping

2 cups strawberries, halved

Make Crust

1. Preheat the oven to 350°F. Coat a 9-inch tart pan with removable bottom with cooking spray and set aside.

2. Place the crumbled graham crackers in a food processor and process until finely ground. Transfer to a medium bowl and stir in the butter-flavored spread and egg white. Coat your hands lightly with cooking spray and press the mixture into the bottom and up the sides of the prepared pan.

3. Bake 8 to 10 minutes or until the crust is lightly browned (small cracks may appear). Cool completely on a wire rack.

Make Filling

1. Combine the milk, egg yolk, no-calorie sweetener, sugar, cornstarch, and salt in a medium heavy-bottomed saucepan and whisk until the cornstarch dissolves. Cook over medium heat, whisking constantly, about 6 minutes or until the mixture comes to a boil and thickens.

2. Remove from the heat and whisk in the preserves and cream cheese. Transfer to a medium bowl and cover the surface of the filling with plastic wrap to prevent a skin from forming. Cool to room temperature and stir in the vanilla. Spoon into the prepared crust. Cover and refrigerate 2 hours or until firm. Arrange the strawberries cut side down on tart just before serving.

Exchanges: 2 Carbohydrate • 1/2 Fat
Calories 163, Calories from Fat 39, Total Fat 4 g, Saturated Fat 1 g, Cholesterol 25 mg, Sodium 170 mg, Total Carbohydrate 27 g, Dietary Fiber 1 g, Sugars 15 g, Protein 4 g.

Mango–Lime Tart

Makes 10 servings • Serving size: 1 slice

The tropical flavors of this tart are reminiscent of Key lime pie. By all means, use real
Key limes if you have access to them—they'll make this cool-you-down pie taste even better.

Crust

9 low-fat graham crackers, crumbled
(use 9 whole rectangles)

1 teaspoon ground ginger (optional)

2 tablespoons 67% vegetable oil butter-
flavored spread, melted and cooled

1 egg white

Filling

1 cup fat-free milk

1/2 cup fat-free sweetened condensed milk

1/2 cup fresh lime juice

2 egg yolks

1/2 cup granular no-calorie sweetener

1/4 cup cornstarch

1/4 teaspoon salt

2 tablespoons reduced-fat sour cream

1 tablespoon fresh grated lime zest

Topping

1 medium ripe mango, peeled and
thinly sliced

Make Crust

1. Preheat the oven to 350°F. Coat a 9-inch tart pan with removable bottom with cooking spray and set aside.

2. Place the crumbled graham crackers and ginger, if using, in a food processor and process until finely ground. Transfer to a medium bowl and stir in the butter-flavored spread and egg white. Coat your hands lightly with cooking spray and press the mixture into the bottom and up the sides of the prepared pan.

3. Bake 8 to 10 minutes or until the crust is lightly browned (small cracks may appear). Cool completely on a wire rack.

Make Filling

1. Combine the fat-free milk, condensed milk, lime juice, egg yolks, no-calorie sweetener, cornstarch, and salt in a medium heavy-bottomed saucepan and whisk until the cornstarch dissolves. Cook over medium heat, whisking constantly, about 6 minutes or until the mixture comes to a boil and thickens.

2. Remove from the heat and stir in the sour cream and lime zest. Transfer to a medium bowl and cover the surface of the filling with plastic wrap to prevent a skin from forming. Cool to room temperature and spoon into the prepared crust. Cover and refrigerate 2 hours or until firm. Top with mango slices just before serving.

Exchanges: 2 Carbohydrate • 1/2 Fat
Calories 176, Calories from Fat 37, Total Fat 4 g, Saturated Fat 1 g, Cholesterol 44 mg, Sodium 202 mg, Total Carbohydrate 31 g, Dietary Fiber 1 g, Sugars 19 g, Protein 4 g.

BLUEBERRY–LEMON CURD TART

Makes 10 servings • Serving size: 1 slice

A slice of this chilly tart will cool you off on a hot summer day.
Substitute other berries for the blueberries, or serve it plain.

Crust

9 low-fat graham crackers, crumbled
(use 9 whole rectangles)

2 tablespoons 67% vegetable oil butter-
flavored spread, melted and cooled

1 egg white

Filling

1 1/2 cups water

1/2 cup fresh lemon juice

1 egg yolk

1 cup granular no-calorie sweetener

1/4 cup granulated sugar

1/4 cup cornstarch

Pinch of salt

1/4 cup reduced-fat sour cream

1 tablespoon fresh grated lemon zest

Topping

1 1/2 cups fresh blueberries

Make Crust

1. Preheat the oven to 350°F. Coat a 9-inch tart pan with removable bottom with cooking spray and set aside.

2. Place the crumbled graham crackers in a food processor and process until finely ground. Transfer to a medium bowl and stir in the butter-flavored spread and egg white. Coat your hands lightly with cooking spray and press the mixture into the bottom and up the sides of the prepared pan.

3. Bake 8 to 10 minutes or until the crust is lightly browned (small cracks may appear). Cool completely on a wire rack.

Make Filling

1. Combine the water, lemon juice, egg yolk, no-calorie sweetener, sugar, cornstarch, and salt in a large heavy-bottomed saucepan and whisk until the cornstarch dissolves. Cook over medium heat, whisking constantly, about 6 minutes or until the mixture comes to a boil and thickens.

2. Remove from the heat and stir in the sour cream and lemon zest. Transfer to a medium bowl and cover the surface of the filling with plastic wrap to prevent a skin from forming. Cool to room temperature.

3. Spoon the filling into the prepared crust. Top with blueberries, cover, and refrigerate 2 hours or until firm.

Exchanges: 1 1/2 Carbohydrate • 1/2 Fat
Calories 143, Calories from Fat 35, Total Fat 4 g, Saturated Fat 1 g, Cholesterol 24 mg, Sodium 133 mg, Total Carbohydrate 26 g, Dietary Fiber 1 g, Sugars 14 g, Protein 2 g.

Almond Tart with Poached Peaches

Makes 10 servings • Serving size: 1 slice

Peaches and almonds are a classic flavor pairing, and this dessert showcases the duo perfectly. It requires a bit of work, but the luscious flavor and beauty of this tart make it worth the effort.

Crust

9 low-fat graham crackers, crumbled (use 9 whole rectangles)

1/3 cup sliced almonds

2 tablespoons 67% vegetable oil butter-flavored spread, melted and cooled

1 egg white

Filling

2 cups 1% low-fat milk

1 egg yolk

2/3 cup granular no-calorie sweetener

1/4 cup granulated sugar

1/4 cup cornstarch

Pinch of salt

1 teaspoon almond extract

Topping

1/4 cup water

3 tablespoons granulated sugar

6 medium peaches, peeled, pitted, and halved

2 tablespoons sliced almonds

Make Crust

1. Preheat the oven to 350°F. Coat a 9-inch tart pan with removable bottom with cooking spray and set aside.

2. Place the crumbled graham crackers and almonds in a food processor and process until finely ground. Transfer to a medium bowl and stir in the butter-flavored spread and egg white. Coat your hands lightly with cooking spray and press the mixture into the bottom and up the sides of the prepared pan.

3. Bake 8 to 10 minutes or until the crust is lightly browned (small cracks may appear). Cool completely on a wire rack.

Make Filling

1. Combine the milk, egg yolk, no-calorie sweetener, sugar, cornstarch, and salt in a medium heavy-bottomed saucepan and whisk until the cornstarch dissolves. Cook over medium heat, whisking constantly, about 6 minutes or until the mixture comes to a boil and thickens.

2. Transfer to a medium bowl and cover the surface of the filling with plastic wrap to prevent a skin from forming. Cool to room temperature. Stir in the almond extract. Spoon into the prepared crust, cover, and refrigerate 2 hours or until firm.

Make Topping

1. Combine the water and sugar in a medium skillet and bring to a boil over medium-high heat. Add the peach halves, cover, reduce heat to low, and simmer 8 to 10 minutes or until the peaches have softened, but not lost their shape. Cool the peaches to room temperature in the cooking liquid.

2. To serve, arrange peaches cut side down on the tart filling using a slotted spoon. Cook the liquid remaining in the skillet over medium high heat for 3 to 5 minutes or until reduced to 1 tablespoon. Drizzle the liquid over the tart, sprinkle with the almonds, and serve immediately.

Exchanges: 2 1/2 Carbohydrate • 1 Fat
Calories 212, Calories from Fat 55, Total Fat 6 g, Saturated Fat 1 g, Cholesterol 24 mg, Sodium 150 mg, Total Carbohydrate 36 g, Dietary Fiber 2 g, Sugars 24 g, Protein 5 g.

Fresh Apricot–Ginger Tart

Makes 10 servings • Serving size: 1 slice

What better way to celebrate the start of summer than with this fabulously flavorful tart made with the season's first apricots? Make it in the afternoon before an outdoor dinner party and serve slices of summer magic under the stars.

Crust

1 cup all-purpose flour

1/2 teaspoon salt

1/2 teaspoon baking powder

1/4 teaspoon baking soda

1/4 cup canola oil

3 tablespoons reduced-fat sour cream

Filling

1/3 cup unsweetened applesauce

2 teaspoons fresh grated ginger

12 small ripe apricots (about 1 1/4 pounds), halved and pitted

3 tablespoons granulated sugar

Make Crust

1. Preheat the oven to 350°F. Coat a 9-inch tart pan with removable bottom with cooking spray and set aside.

2. Combine the flour, salt, baking powder, and baking soda in a medium bowl. Combine the oil and sour cream in a small bowl and whisk until well mixed. Add the oil mixture to the flour mixture and stir until a stiff dough forms. Shape the dough into a disk and place between 2 sheets of waxed paper.

3. Roll the dough to a 12-inch diameter circle. Remove the top layer of waxed paper and place the dough, with waxed paper facing up, into the prepared tart pan. Starting from the edge of the dough, gently remove the waxed paper. Trim the edges of the crust.

Make Filling

1. Combine the applesauce and ginger in a small bowl and stir to mix well. Spread evenly over the bottom of the crust.

2. Arrange the apricots, cut side up, in a single layer in the crust. Sprinkle the apricots with sugar. Place the tart pan on a foil-lined baking sheet. Bake 1 hour to 1 hour and 10 minutes or until the edge of the crust is browned and the apricots are soft. Cool on a wire rack. Serve slightly warm or at room temperature.

Exchanges: 1 1/2 Carbohydrate • 1 Fat
Calories 143, Calories from Fat 55, Total Fat 6 g, Saturated Fat 1 g, Cholesterol 2 mg, Sodium 171 mg, Total Carbohydrate 20 g, Dietary Fiber 2 g, Sugars 10 g, Protein 2 g.

Chocolate-Drizzled Peanut Butter Cake, p 16
Chocolate Crackles, p 199

Fruit-Filled Layer Cake with White Chocolate Frosting, p 44

Dainty Dried Fruit Loaves, p 57
Lemon Surprise Muffins, p 67

Very Berry Raspberry Tart, p 124
Peach Melba Shortcakes, p 72

Apple Pie with Cinnamon
Crunch Topping , p 78

**Warm Summer Fruits with
Sour Cream and Brown Sugar, p 147**

Chocolate Velvet Pudding, p 164
Pumpkin Flan, p 174

Chocolate–Peppermint Ice Cream Cake, p 218

FRESH FIG TART

Makes 10 servings • Serving size: 1 slice

This is the recipe to use if you can't get enough of the short season of fresh figs. A touch of orange in the filling is a nice counterpoint to the sweet figs.

Filling

1/4 cup granulated sugar

1/4 cup granular no-calorie sweetener

1 tablespoon all-purpose flour

1 tablespoon fresh grated orange zest

1 1/2 pounds small ripe fresh figs, stemmed and quartered (about 35 figs)

Crust

1 cup all-purpose flour

1/2 teaspoon salt

1/2 teaspoon baking powder

1/4 teaspoon baking soda

1/4 cup canola oil

3 tablespoons reduced-fat sour cream

Make Filling

1. Combine the sugar, no-calorie sweetener, flour, and orange zest in a large bowl and stir to mix well.
2. Add the figs and toss to coat. Set aside.

Make Crust

1. Preheat the oven to 350°F. Coat a 9-inch tart pan with removable bottom with cooking spray and set aside.
2. Combine the flour, salt, baking powder, and baking soda in a medium bowl. Combine the oil and sour cream in a small bowl and whisk until smooth. Add the oil mixture to the flour mixture and stir until a stiff dough forms. Shape the dough into a disk and place between 2 sheets of waxed paper.
3. Roll the dough to a 12-inch diameter circle. Remove the top layer of waxed paper and place the dough, with waxed paper facing up, into the prepared tart pan. Starting from the edge of the dough, gently remove the waxed paper. Trim the edges of the crust.
4. Arrange the figs in the prepared crust. Place the tart pan on a foil-lined baking sheet. Bake 55 to 60 minutes or until the edge of the crust is browned and the figs are soft. Cool on a wire rack. Serve slightly warm or at room temperature.

Exchanges: 2 Carbohydrate • 1 Fat
Calories 175, Calories from Fat 55, Total Fat 6 g, Saturated Fat 1 g, Cholesterol 2 mg, Sodium 171 mg, Total Carbohydrate 29 g, Dietary Fiber 3 g, Sugars 11 g, Protein 2 g.

Blackberry–Pecan Tart

Makes 10 servings • Serving size: 1 slice

Grape juice makes a jewel-toned complement to succulent blackberries in this stunning tart. Use only fresh berries, as frozen ones won't hold their shape.

Crust

9 low-fat graham crackers, crumbled (use 9 whole rectangles)

1/3 cup chopped pecans

2 tablespoons 67% vegetable oil butter-flavored spread, melted and cooled

1 egg white

Filling

2 cups unsweetened purple grape juice

1/4 cup granular no-calorie sweetener

3 tablespoons cornstarch

2 tablespoons granulated sugar

2 cups fresh blackberries

Make Crust

1. Preheat the oven to 350°F. Coat a 9-inch tart pan with removable bottom with cooking spray and set aside.

2. Place the crumbled graham crackers and pecans in a food processor and process until finely ground. Transfer to a medium bowl and stir in the butter-flavored spread and egg white. Coat your hands lightly with cooking spray and press the mixture into the bottom and up the sides of the prepared pan.

3. Place the tart pan on a baking sheet and bake 8 to 10 minutes or until the crust is lightly browned (small cracks may appear). Cool completely on a wire rack.

Make Filling

1. Combine the grape juice, no-calorie sweetener, cornstarch, and sugar in a medium heavy-bottomed saucepan and stir until the cornstarch dissolves. Cook over medium heat, stirring constantly, about 6 minutes or until the mixture comes to a boil and thickens.

2. Transfer to a large bowl and cover the surface of the filling with plastic wrap to prevent a skin from forming. Let stand 45 minutes or until almost cool. Add the blackberries and stir gently to combine.

3. Pour the filling into the crust, place a sheet of plastic wrap on the surface of the filling, and refrigerate 2 hours or until firm.

Exchanges: 2 Carbohydrate • 1/2 Fat
Calories 166, Calories from Fat 51, Total Fat 6 g, Saturated Fat 1 g, Cholesterol 0 mg, Sodium 111 mg, Total Carbohydrate 28 g, Dietary Fiber 2 g, Sugars 16 g, Protein 2 g.

Very Berry Raspberry Tart

Makes 10 servings • Serving size: 1 slice

This tart's so elegant and easy, you'll make it all summer long.

Crust

1 cup all-purpose flour

1/2 teaspoon salt

1/2 teaspoon baking powder

1/4 teaspoon baking soda

1/4 cup canola oil

3 tablespoons reduced-fat sour cream

Filling

4 cups fresh raspberries

1/2 cup sugar-free red raspberry preserves

1/4 cup water

Make Crust

1. Preheat the oven to 400°F. Coat a 9-inch tart pan with removable bottom with cooking spray and set aside.

2. Combine the flour, salt, baking powder, and baking soda in a medium bowl. Combine the oil and sour cream in a small bowl and whisk until well mixed. Add the oil mixture to the flour mixture and stir until a stiff dough forms. Shape the dough into a disk and place between 2 sheets of waxed paper.

3. Roll the dough to a 12-inch diameter circle. Remove the top layer of waxed paper and place the dough, with waxed paper facing up, into the prepared pan. Starting from the edge of the dough, gently remove the waxed paper. Trim the edges of the crust and prick the bottom all over with a fork. Bake 10 to 12 minutes or until the crust is lightly browned. Cool completely on a wire rack.

Make Filling

1. Place the raspberries in a large bowl. Place a fine mesh sieve in the bowl over the raspberries.

2. Combine the preserves and water in a small saucepan. Cook over medium heat, stirring constantly, until the preserves melt. Pour the mixture through the sieve over the raspberries, pressing with a spatula to extract all liquid. Discard the solids.

3. Gently stir the raspberries to coat with the preserves mixture. Spoon into the prepared crust. Cover and refrigerate 2 hours or until firm.

Exchanges: 1 Carbohydrate • 1 Fat
Calories 132, Calories from Fat 56, Total Fat 6 g, Saturated Fat 1 g, Cholesterol 2 mg, Sodium 170 mg, Total Carbohydrate 18 g, Dietary Fiber 4 g, Sugars 3 g, Protein 2 g.

Apple–Currant Tarte Tatin

Makes 8 servings • Serving size: 1 slice

Tarte Tatin is a classic French dessert that's baked upside down—the apples go on the bottom and the crust on top. When inverted onto a plate for serving, the tender apples and caramelized sugar sit atop a perfectly crisp crust. Arranging the apples in concentric circles makes a pretty presentation, but if you're in a hurry, just put them in the skillet randomly.

Filling

1 tablespoon 67% vegetable oil butter-flavored spread

3 tablespoons granulated sugar, divided use

1 1/2 tablespoons all-purpose flour

3/4 teaspoon ground cinnamon

Pinch of salt

4 medium Granny Smith apples (about 1 1/2 pounds) peeled, cored, and sliced into 1/4-inch-thick slices (about 5 cups)

2 tablespoons dried currants

Crust

1 cup all-purpose flour

1/2 teaspoon salt

1/2 teaspoon baking powder

1/4 teaspoon baking soda

1/4 cup canola oil

3 tablespoons reduced-fat sour cream

Make Filling

1. Preheat the oven to 375°F.

2. Melt the butter-flavored spread in a 10-inch ovenproof skillet. Remove from the heat and coat the sides of the skillet with cooking spray. Sprinkle 2 tablespoons of the sugar evenly in the bottom of the skillet.

3. Combine the flour, cinnamon, and salt in a large bowl and stir to mix well. Add the apples and toss to coat. Arrange the apples slices in concentric circles in the bottom of the skillet. Sprinkle with the currants and remaining 1 tablespoon sugar. Set aside.

Make Crust

1. Combine the flour, salt, baking powder, and baking soda in a medium bowl. Combine the oil and sour cream in a small bowl and whisk until well mixed. Add the oil mixture to the flour mixture and stir until a stiff dough forms. Shape the dough into a disk and place between 2 sheets of waxed paper.

2. Roll the dough to a 12-inch diameter circle. Remove the top layer of waxed paper and place the dough, with waxed paper facing up, over the apple mixture in the skillet. Starting from the edge of the dough, gently remove the waxed paper. Gently press the edge of the crust into the apple mixture. Bake 30 to 35 minutes or until the apples are bubbling and the crust is lightly browned. Immediately invert the tart onto a serving platter. Cool 10 minutes before serving. Serve warm.

Exchanges: 2 Carbohydrate • 1 1/2 Fat
Calories 208, Calories from Fat 80, Total Fat 9 g, Saturated Fat 1 g, Cholesterol 2 mg, Sodium 242 mg, Total Carbohydrate 31 g, Dietary Fiber 2 g, Sugars 16 g, Protein 2 g.

Berry Tartlets with Honey Cream

Makes 8 servings • Serving size: 1 tartlet

You can make almost endless variations of these tartlets, since the flavor of the filling depends on the variety of honey you use. And you can use almost any soft fruit instead of the berries—try chopped peaches, nectarines, apricots, or plums.

Crusts

8 frozen phyllo sheets, thawed (9 × 14 inches each)

Filling

1 1/4 cups 1% low-fat milk

1/2 cup honey

1/3 cup cornstarch

1 egg yolk

Pinch of salt

Topping

2 cups fresh blueberries or raspberries

Make Crusts

1. Preheat the oven to 375°F. Coat 8 muffin cups with cooking spray and set aside.

2. Place 1 sheet of phyllo on a work surface and lightly coat with cooking spray. Top with 3 of the remaining phyllo sheets, coating each sheet with cooking spray. Cut stacked phyllo sheets in half lengthwise, then in half crosswise, forming 4 (7 × 4 1/2-inch) rectangles. Fit the dough into the prepared cups, pressing the bottom and sides against the cups and ruffling overhanging edges. Repeat the procedure with the 4 remaining phyllo sheets.

3. Prick the bottom of each phyllo cup several times with a fork. Bake 8 minutes or until crusts are lightly browned.

4. Cool in the pan on a wire rack for 5 minutes. Carefully remove the crusts from the cups and cool completely on the wire rack.

Make Filling

1. Combine the milk, honey, cornstarch, egg yolk, and salt in a medium heavy-bottomed saucepan and whisk until the cornstarch dissolves. Cook over medium heat, whisking constantly, about 6 minutes or until the mixture comes to a boil and thickens.

2. Transfer to a medium bowl and cover the surface of the filling with plastic wrap to prevent a skin from forming. Cool to room temperature. Spoon 3 tablespoons of the filling into each tartlet shell and top evenly with the berries. Serve immediately.

Exchanges: 2 1/2 Carbohydrate
Calories 165, Calories from Fat 15, Total Fat 2 g, Saturated Fat 1 g, Cholesterol 30 mg, Sodium 103 mg, Total Carbohydrate 37 g, Dietary Fiber 1 g, Sugars 23 g, Protein 3 g.

HOLIDAY CRANBERRY TARTS

Makes 6 servings • Serving size: 1 tartlet

There's no need to chill these tarts before serving. To make them a day ahead, store the baked crusts in their pans at room temperature in resealable zip-top bags. Cover and refrigerate the cranberry filling, but bring it to room temperature before spooning into the crusts.

Crusts

9 low-fat graham crackers, crumbled (use 9 whole rectangles)

1/2 teaspoon ground cinnamon

2 tablespoons 67% vegetable oil butter-flavored spread, melted and cooled

1 egg white

Filling

1 (12-ounce) bag fresh cranberries

1/2 cup granulated sugar

1/2 cup granular no-calorie sweetener

2 tablespoons water

2 teaspoons fresh grated orange zest

Make Crusts

1. Preheat the oven to 350°F. Coat 6 (4-inch) tartlet pans with removable bottoms with cooking spray and set aside.

2. Place crumbled graham crackers and cinnamon in a food processor and process until finely ground. Transfer to a medium bowl and stir in the butter-flavored spread and egg white. Coat your hands lightly with cooking spray and press about 1/4 cup of the graham cracker mixture into the bottom and up the sides of each of the prepared pans.

3. Place the tart pans on a baking sheet and bake 10 to 12 minutes or until the crusts are lightly browned (small cracks may appear). Cool completely on a wire rack.

Make Filling

1. Combine the cranberries, sugar, no-calorie sweetener, and water in a medium saucepan. Cook over medium-high heat, stirring constantly, 5 minutes or until the cranberries pop. Remove from the heat and stir in the orange zest.

2. Cool the filling and spoon into the prepared crusts. The tartlets are best served within 2 hours of assembling.

Exchanges: 3 Carbohydrate • 1/2 Fat
Calories 223, Calories from Fat 43, Total Fat 5 g, Saturated Fat 1 g, Cholesterol 0 mg, Sodium 183 mg, Total Carbohydrate 45 g, Dietary Fiber 3 g, Sugars 29 g, Protein 2 g.

Fruity Desserts

SOUTHERN PEACH AND BLACKBERRY CRUMBLE

Makes 8 servings • Serving size: 1/2 cup

A perfect ending to a summer supper or brunch, this homey dessert showcases peaches, blackberries, pecans, and cornmeal—all staples of Southern cuisine.

6 large ripe peaches (about 1 3/4 pounds), peeled, pitted, and sliced, or 3 1/2 cups unsweetened frozen sliced peaches, thawed

2 cups fresh blackberries or unsweetened frozen blackberries, unthawed

2 tablespoons all-purpose flour

1 tablespoon fresh grated lemon zest

1/4 cup light brown sugar

3 tablespoons yellow cornmeal (not cornmeal mix)

1/2 teaspoon ground cinnamon

3 tablespoons 67% vegetable oil butter-flavored spread, chilled

1/4 cup chopped pecans

1. Preheat the oven to 350°F. Coat an 8 × 8-inch glass baking dish with cooking spray and set aside.

2. Combine the peaches, blackberries, flour, and lemon zest in a large bowl and toss to combine. Spoon into prepared dish.

3. Combine the brown sugar, cornmeal, cinnamon, and butter-flavored spread in a medium bowl. Blend together using a pastry blender or your fingertips until the butter-flavored spread is uniformly incorporated. Stir in the pecans. Sprinkle evenly over the peach mixture.

4. Bake 25 to 30 minutes or until the topping is lightly browned and the fruit is bubbly around the edges. Let stand 10 minutes before serving. Serve warm.

Exchanges: 1 1/2 Carbohydrate • 1 Fat
Calories 155, Calories from Fat 58, Total Fat 6 g, Saturated Fat 1 g, Cholesterol 0 mg, Sodium 37 mg, Total Carbohydrate 24 g, Dietary Fiber 4 g, Sugars 17 g, Protein 2 g.

PEAK OF SUMMER FRUIT CRUMBLE

Makes 8 servings • Serving size: 1/2 cup

Almond paste stands in for the butter in the topping for this crumble,
cutting saturated fat and adding great flavor. Make this in June and July
when apricots and cherries are both at their best.

12 small apricots
(about 1 1/4 pounds),
pitted and sliced

2 cups fresh sweet
cherries, pitted, or
frozen, unsweetened
cherries, thawed

1/4 cup all-purpose flour

1/4 cup light brown sugar

1/4 cup almond paste,
crumbled

2 tablespoons 67% vegetable
oil butter-flavored spread

1/4 cup slivered almonds

1. Preheat the oven to 350°F. Coat an 8 × 8-inch glass baking dish with cooking spray. Place the apricots and cherries in the prepared dish.

2. Combine the flour, brown sugar, almond paste, and butter-flavored spread in a medium bowl. Blend together using a pastry blender or your fingertips until the butter-flavored spread is uniformly incorporated. Stir in the almonds. Sprinkle evenly over the apricot mixture.

3. Bake 25 to 30 minutes or until the topping is lightly browned and the fruit is bubbly around the edges. Let stand 10 minutes before serving. Serve warm.

Exchanges: 2 Carbohydrate • 1 Fat
Calories 175, Calories from Fat 64, Total Fat 7 g, Saturated Fat 1 g, Cholesterol 0 mg,
Sodium 27 mg, Total Carbohydrate 27 g, Dietary Fiber 3 g, Sugars 21 g, Protein 3 g.

Autumn Pear and Cranberry Crumble

Makes 8 servings • Serving size: 1 slice

You'll make this simple crumble again and again when pears and fresh cranberries show up in the markets. Tender fruit is suspended in an airy orange-spiked batter and topped with a crunchy crumb topping. It's perfect with brunch or as dessert after a casual supper.

Cake

1 cup all-purpose flour

1/2 cup no-calorie sweetener

2 tablespoons granulated sugar

1 teaspoon baking powder

1/4 teaspoon salt

1/4 cup canola oil

1/4 cup fresh-squeezed orange juice

1 large egg

1 teaspoon almond extract

1 tablespoon fresh grated orange zest

3 large ripe pears (about 1 1/4 pounds), peeled, cored, and cut into 1/2-inch pieces (about 2 1/2 cups)

1 cup fresh cranberries or frozen cranberries, unthawed

Topping

1/4 cup light brown sugar

1/4 cup old-fashioned (not quick-cooking) oats

1 1/2 tablespoons 67% vegetable oil butter-flavored spread, at room temperature

1/4 cup sliced almonds

Make Cake

1. Preheat the oven to 350°F. Coat a 9 1/2-inch deep-dish glass pie plate with cooking spray and set aside.

2. Combine the flour, no-calorie sweetener, sugar, baking powder, and salt in a large bowl and whisk to mix well. Set aside.

3. Combine the oil, orange juice, egg, and almond extract in a medium bowl and whisk until smooth. Stir in the orange zest. Add the oil mixture to the flour mixture and stir just until moistened. Stir in the pears and cranberries. Spoon the batter into the prepared pie plate.

Make Topping

1. Combine the brown sugar and oats in a medium bowl. Add the butter-flavored spread and blend into the dry ingredients using a pastry blender or your fingertips until the spread is uniformly incorporated. Stir in the almonds and sprinkle mixture over the batter.

2. Bake 45 to 50 minutes or until the topping is lightly browned. Cool in the pan on a wire rack for 10 minutes. Let stand 10 minutes before serving. Serve warm.

Exchanges: 2 1/2 Carbohydrate • 1 Fat
Calories 236, Calories from Fat 69, Total Fat 8 g, Saturated Fat 1 g, Cholesterol 26 mg, Sodium 128 mg, Total Carbohydrate 40 g, Dietary Fiber 3 g, Sugars 24 g, Protein 3 g.

Biscuit-Topped Country Apple Cobbler

Makes 8 servings • Serving size: 1/2 cup

Simple and homey, this dessert is what to serve after a Sunday supper in October. If your carb and calorie budget allows, enjoy it with a scoop of fat-free, no-sugar-added vanilla ice cream.

Fruit Filling

6 medium Granny Smith apples (about 2 1/4 pounds) peeled, cored, and sliced into 1/4-inch-thick slices (about 7 cups)

2 teaspoons fresh grated lemon zest

2 tablespoons fresh lemon juice

1/4 cup granulated sugar

1/4 teaspoon ground ginger

1/4 teaspoon ground nutmeg

1/4 teaspoon ground cinnamon

Biscuit Topping

1 cup all-purpose flour

1 tablespoon granulated sugar

1 teaspoon baking powder

1/2 teaspoon baking soda

1/4 teaspoon salt

1 tablespoon 67% vegetable oil butter-flavored spread

1/2 cup low-fat buttermilk

Make Filling

1. Preheat the oven to 350°F. Coat an 11 × 7-inch glass baking dish with cooking spray and set aside.

2. Place the apples in a large bowl, add the lemon zest and lemon juice, and toss to coat. Combine the sugar, ginger, nutmeg, and cinnamon in a small bowl and stir to mix well. Add the sugar mixture to the apples and toss to combine. Place the apple mixture in the prepared baking dish.

Make Topping

1. Combine the flour, sugar, baking powder, baking soda, and salt in a large bowl. Add the butter-flavored spread and blend into dry ingredients using a pastry blender or your fingertips until the spread is uniformly incorporated. Add the buttermilk and stir just until moistened. Drop the batter by spoonfuls over the apple mixture.

2. Bake for 35 to 40 minutes or until the biscuits are well-browned and the apples are tender. Let stand 10 minutes before serving. Serve warm.

Exchanges: 2 Carbohydrate
Calories 156, Calories from Fat 16, Total Fat 2 g, Saturated Fat 1 g, Cholesterol 1 mg, Sodium 225 mg, Total Carbohydrate 34 g, Dietary Fiber 2 g, Sugars 20 g, Protein 2 g.

Gingerbread–Apple Cobbler

Makes 8 servings • Serving size: 1/2 cup

A step above the average apple cobbler, this version tops fresh apple slices with a spicy gingerbread batter. Generous measures of ground ginger and black pepper give it a sophisticated flavor adults will love.

Fruit Filling

4 medium Granny Smith apples (about 1 1/2 pounds), peeled, cored, and sliced into 1/4-inch-thick slices (about 6 cups)

1/3 cup raisins

2 teaspoons fresh grated lemon zest

2 tablespoons fresh lemon juice

1/2 teaspoon ground cinnamon

Gingerbread Topping

1/2 cup granular no-calorie sweetener

1/2 cup molasses

1/4 cup canola oil

1/4 cup low-fat buttermilk

1 large egg

1/2 cup all-purpose flour

1/2 cup whole wheat flour

1 tablespoon ground ginger

1/2 teaspoon baking powder

1/2 teaspoon baking soda

1/4 teaspoon ground allspice

1/4 teaspoon ground cloves

1/4 teaspoon salt

1/4 teaspoon fresh ground black pepper

Make Filling

1. Preheat the oven to 350°F. Coat an 8 × 8-inch glass baking dish with cooking spray and set aside.

2. Place the apples and raisins in a large bowl. Add the lemon zest, lemon juice, and cinnamon and toss to combine. Spoon the apple mixture into the prepared pan and bake 15 minutes.

Make Topping

1. Meanwhile, combine the no-calorie sweetener, molasses, oil, buttermilk, and egg in a medium bowl and whisk until the mixture is smooth.

2. Combine the all-purpose flour, whole wheat flour, ginger, baking powder, baking soda, allspice, cloves, salt, and pepper in a medium bowl and whisk to mix well. Add the no-calorie sweetener mixture to the flour mixture and stir just until moistened. Remove the cobbler from the oven and spoon the batter evenly over the apples. Bake 20 to 25 minutes longer or until the topping is lightly browned around the edges and the apples are tender. Let stand 10 minutes before serving. Serve warm.

Exchanges: 3 Carbohydrate • 1 Fat
Calories 241, Calories from Fat 72, Total Fat 8 g, Saturated Fat 1 g, Cholesterol 27 mg, Sodium 200 mg, Total Carbohydrate 42 g, Dietary Fiber 3 g, Sugars 26 g, Protein 3 g.

CHERRY–ORANGE COBBLER

Makes 10 servings • Serving size: 1/2 cup

As this super-fruity cobbler bakes, it perfumes the kitchen with intoxicating aroma.
Serve it for dessert at a midsummer barbecue.

2 large navel or
Valencia oranges

6 cups fresh sweet cherries,
pitted or unsweetened
frozen cherries, thawed

3/4 cup low-fat buttermilk

2 tablespoons canola oil

1 large egg

1 cup all-purpose flour

1/4 cup granulated sugar

1/4 cup granular no-calorie
sweetener

1 teaspoon baking powder

1/2 teaspoon baking soda

1/4 teaspoon salt

1. Preheat the oven to 350°F. Coat a 9 1/2-inch deep-dish glass pie plate with cooking spray and set aside. Grate 2 teaspoons zest from the oranges and place in a medium bowl. Set aside.

2. Cut a thin slice from the top and bottom of each of the oranges, exposing the flesh. Stand each fruit upright, and using a sharp knife, thickly cut off the peel, following the contour of the fruit and removing all the white pith and membrane. Holding the fruit over a bowl, carefully cut along both sides of each section to free it from the membrane. Discard any seeds and let the sections fall into the bowl. Using two forks, separate the sections into small pieces. Add the cherries and stir to combine. Transfer to the prepared pie plate.

3. Add the buttermilk, oil, and egg to the reserved orange zest and whisk to mix well. Combine the flour, sugar, no-calorie sweetener, baking powder, baking soda, and salt in a medium bowl and whisk to mix well. Stir in the buttermilk mixture. Spoon the batter over the cherry mixture, leaving some of the cherries uncovered. Bake 25 to 30 minutes or until the topping is lightly browned and the fruit is bubbly around the edges. Let stand 10 minutes before serving. Serve warm.

Exchanges: 2 Carbohydrate • 1/2 Fat

Calories 183, Calories from Fat 40, Total Fat 4 g, Saturated Fat 1 g, Cholesterol 22 mg, Sodium 184 mg, Total Carbohydrate 34 g, Dietary Fiber 3 g, Sugars 22 g, Protein 4 g.

SUMMER BERRY COBBLER

Makes 8 servings • Serving size: 1/2 cup

There is no flour added to the fruit in this cobbler, but if you'd like the juices to be thickened a little, toss the berries with a tablespoon of flour before placing them in the baking dish. It's wonderful either way.

2 cups fresh blackberries

2 cups fresh raspberries

2 cups fresh blueberries

1 cup all-purpose flour

1 teaspoon baking powder

1/2 teaspoon baking soda

Pinch of salt

2/3 cup low-fat buttermilk

2 tablespoons canola oil

1 large egg

3 tablespoons granulated sugar

3 tablespoons granular no-calorie sweetener

1 teaspoon vanilla extract

2 teaspoons fresh grated lemon zest

1. Preheat the oven to 350°F. Coat an 8 × 8-inch glass baking dish with cooking spray and set aside.

2. Combine the blackberries, raspberries, and blueberries in a large bowl and toss gently to combine. Spoon into the prepared dish.

3. Combine the flour, baking powder, baking soda and salt in a medium bowl and whisk to mix well. Combine the buttermilk, oil, egg, sugar, no-calorie sweetener, and vanilla in a medium bowl and whisk to mix well. Stir in the lemon zest. Add the buttermilk mixture to the flour mixture and stir just until moistened (the batter will be lumpy). Spoon over the berries, leaving some of the berries uncovered.

4. Bake 25 to 30 minutes or until the topping is lightly browned and the fruit is bubbly around the edges. Let stand 10 minutes before serving. Serve warm.

Exchanges: 2 Carbohydrate • 1 Fat
Calories 182, Calories from Fat 44, Total Fat 5 g, Saturated Fat 1 g, Cholesterol 27 mg, Sodium 173 mg, Total Carbohydrate 32 g, Dietary Fiber 5 g, Sugars 14 g, Protein 4 g.

Pineapple–Mango Gingersnap Crisp

Makes 8 servings • Serving size: 1/2 cup

Fresh lime zest and grated ginger give this simple crumble amazing flavor, and gingersnap pieces add crunch. Serve it as a dessert for a Mexican or Caribbean-themed dinner.

3 cups fresh pineapple cubes (1-inch cubes)

2 cups fresh mango cubes (1-inch cubes)

1 tablespoon fresh grated lime zest

1 tablespoon fresh lime juice

2 teaspoons grated fresh ginger

3 tablespoons all-purpose flour

2 tablespoons light brown sugar

8 gingersnap cookies, finely crushed (about 1/2 cup)

2 tablespoons 67% vegetable oil butter-flavored spread, chilled

1. Preheat the oven to 350°F. Coat an 8 × 8-inch glass baking dish with cooking spray and set aside.

2. Combine the pineapple, mango, lime zest, lime juice, and ginger in a large bowl and toss to combine. Combine the flour and the brown sugar in a small bowl and stir to mix well. Add the flour mixture to the pineapple mixture and toss to mix well. Spoon into the prepared dish.

3. Combine the crushed gingersnaps and the butter-flavored spread in a medium bowl. Blend together using a pastry blender or your fingertips until the butter-flavored spread is uniformly incorporated. Sprinkle evenly over the pineapple mixture.

4. Bake 35 to 40 minutes or until the topping is lightly browned and the fruit is bubbly around the edges. Let stand 10 minutes before serving. Serve warm.

Exchanges: 1 1/2 Carbohydrate • 1/2 Fat
Calories 132, Calories from Fat 29, Total Fat 3 g, Saturated Fat 1 g, Cholesterol 0 mg, Sodium 71 mg, Total Carbohydrate 26 g, Dietary Fiber 2 g, Sugars 17 g, Protein 1 g.

Strawberry–Rhubarb Crisp with Almond Crunch Topping

Makes 6 servings • Serving size: 1/2 cup

If you've never tried rhubarb, this recipe is a delicious introduction. Be sure to remove any green leaves from the top of the rhubarb—they contain oxalic acid, which can be toxic.

Filling

1/2 cup granular no-calorie sweetener

2 tablespoons all-purpose flour

2 teaspoons fresh grated orange zest

1 pound fresh rhubarb, cut into 1/2-inch slices (about 3 cups)

1 pint fresh strawberries, halved

Topping

1/4 cup light brown sugar

1/4 cup old-fashioned (not quick-cooking) oats

1/2 teaspoon ground nutmeg

1 1/2 tablespoons 67% vegetable oil butter-flavored spread, at room temperature

1/4 cup slivered almonds

Make Filling

1. Preheat the oven to 350°F. Coat an 8 × 8-inch glass baking dish with cooking spray and set aside.

2. Combine the no-calorie sweetener, flour, and orange zest in a medium bowl and stir to mix well. Add the rhubarb and strawberries and toss to coat. Spoon into the prepared dish.

Make Topping

1. Combine the brown sugar, oats, and nutmeg in a medium bowl. Add the butter-flavored spread and blend into dry ingredients using a pastry blender or your fingertips until the spread is uniformly incorporated. Stir in the almonds and sprinkle over the fruit mixture.

2. Bake 25 to 30 minutes or until the topping is lightly browned and the fruit is bubbly around the edges. Let stand 10 minutes before serving. Serve warm.

Exchanges: 1 1/2 Carbohydrate • 1 Fat
Calories 146, Calories from Fat 52, Total Fat 6 g, Saturated Fat 1 g, Cholesterol 0 mg, Sodium 29 mg, Total Carbohydrate 22 g, Dietary Fiber 3 g, Sugars 14 g, Protein 3 g.

Granny Bartlett Bran Betty

Makes 8 servings • Serving size: 1/2 cup

Lightly spiced slices of sweet apples and pears are layered with a wholesome blend of bran and whole wheat bread crumbs. Use purchased whole wheat crumbs or make your own.

Filling

3 medium Granny Smith apples (about 1 1/4 pounds), peeled, cored, and sliced into 1/4-inch-thick slices

2 medium ripe Bartlett pears (about 1 1/4 pounds), peeled, cored, and sliced into 1/4-inch-thick slices

1 tablespoon fresh lemon juice

2 tablespoons light brown sugar

1/2 teaspoon ground cinnamon

1/4 teaspoon ground nutmeg

1/4 teaspoon salt

Topping

1/4 cup unprocessed wheat bran

1/4 cup whole wheat bread crumbs

2 tablespoons light brown sugar

2 tablespoons 67% vegetable oil butter-flavored spread, chilled

Make Filling

1. Preheat the oven to 350°F. Coat an 8 × 8-inch glass baking dish with cooking spray and set aside.

2. Combine the apples, pears, and lemon juice in a large bowl and toss to coat. Combine the brown sugar, cinnamon, nutmeg, and salt in a small bowl and stir to mix well. Add the brown sugar mixture to the apple mixture and toss to combine. Set aside.

Make Topping

1. Combine the bran, bread crumbs, and brown sugar in a medium bowl. Add the butter-flavored spread and blend into dry ingredients using a pastry blender or your fingertips until the spread is uniformly incorporated.

2. Place half of the fruit mixture in the prepared baking dish. Top with half of the bran mixture. Place the remaining fruit mixture over the bran mixture. Sprinkle with the remaining bran mixture.

3. Bake 35 to 40 minutes or until the topping is lightly browned and the fruit is bubbly around the edges. Let stand 10 minutes before serving. Serve warm.

Exchanges: 2 Carbohydrate

Calories 137, Calories from Fat 26, Total Fat 3 g, Saturated Fat 1 g, Cholesterol 0 mg, Sodium 123 mg, Total Carbohydrate 30 g, Dietary Fiber 4 g, Sugars 21 g, Protein 1 g.

HONEY ROASTED NECTARINES WITH YOGURT CREAM

Makes 8 servings • Serving size: 2 nectarine halves with 2 tablespoons yogurt mixture

The Yogurt Cream served with these simply roasted nectarines is endlessly versatile for topping fresh fruit, a plain cake, or a fruit pie. Experiment with flavorings other than honey. Try adding 1/4 cup granular no-calorie sweetener and 1 teaspoon vanilla extract, 1/4 cup no-sugar-added fruit preserves, or 1/4 cup mashed raspberries or blackberries to 1 cup of drained yogurt.

2 cups plain low-fat yogurt

8 medium ripe nectarines (about 1 1/2 pounds), halved and pitted

3 tablespoons honey, divided use

1. Line a sieve or a colander with several thicknesses of cheesecloth or with a coffee filter and set over a bowl. Spoon the yogurt into the sieve, cover, and refrigerate overnight.

2. Preheat the oven to 375°F. Coat a roasting pan with cooking spray and set aside.

3. Combine the nectarines and 1 tablespoon of the honey in a large bowl and toss to coat. Place the nectarines cut side down in a single layer in prepared pan. Bake 12 to 15 minutes or until nectarines are softened.

4. Combine the drained yogurt and the remaining 2 tablespoons honey in a medium bowl and stir to mix well. Serve the Yogurt Cream with the warm nectarines.

Exchanges: 1 Carbohydrate
Calories 89, Calories from Fat 9, Total Fat 1 g, Saturated Fat 1 g, Cholesterol 3 mg, Sodium 34 mg, Total Carbohydrate 18 g, Dietary Fiber 1 g, Sugars 14 g, Protein 4 g.

Warm Summer Fruits with Sour Cream and Brown Sugar

Makes 6 servings • Serving size: 1/2 cup

Broiling the fruits gives off their juices, which mix with the sour cream to make a luscious, creamy sauce. Substituting nectarines or apricots for the peaches and blackberries or raspberries for the blueberries gives equally delicious results.

4 medium ripe peaches, peeled, pitted, and sliced, or 3 cups frozen unsweetened peach slices, thawed

1 cup fresh blueberries or frozen unsweetened blueberries, thawed

1/4 cup reduced-fat sour cream

1 tablespoon fat-free milk

1 teaspoon vanilla extract

2 tablespoons light brown sugar

1. Place the broiler rack 4 inches from the heat source. Preheat the broiler.

2. Place the peaches and blueberries in a 2-quart flameproof (not glass) baking dish and toss to combine.

3. Combine the sour cream, milk, and vanilla in a small bowl and stir to mix well. Spoon the sour cream mixture over the fruit and sprinkle with brown sugar.

4. Broil, carefully turning pan if necessary, for 4 to 5 minutes or until the fruit is warmed and the sugar is lightly browned. Serve immediately.

Exchanges: 1 Carbohydrate
Calories 86, Calories from Fat 10, Total Fat 1 g, Saturated Fat 1 g, Cholesterol 4 mg, Sodium 12 mg, Total Carbohydrate 18 g, Dietary Fiber 2 g, Sugars 16 g, Protein 2 g.

WINE AND SPICE SOAKED FIGS

Makes 10 servings • Serving size: 2 figs with 1 teaspoon glaze

Serve these accompanied with simple drained yogurt, or dress them up with crumbled blue cheese and toasted walnuts. Cellophane-wrapped boxes tend to flatten dried figs. If yours are less than perfect, gently press them back into teardrop shapes before baking.

1 pound whole dried Calimyrna figs

Peel from one large lemon, yellow part only, removed with a vegetable peeler in strips

Peel from one large orange, orange part only, removed with a vegetable peeler in strips

1 (3-inch) cinnamon stick

1 1/2 cups dry red wine

1/3 cup granulated sugar

1. Preheat the oven to 350°F.

2. Place the figs, lemon peel, orange peel, and cinnamon stick in a single layer in an 11 × 7-inch glass baking dish.

3. Combine the wine and sugar in a small saucepan and heat to boiling. Pour over the figs. Cover and bake 1 hour and 15 minutes to 1 hour and 30 minutes or until the figs are plumped and the sauce is thickened.

4. Cool the figs in the cooking liquid. The figs may be kept in an airtight container and stored in the refrigerator for 4 days. Bring to room temperature and remove the cinnamon stick before serving.

Exchanges: 2 1/2 Carbohydrate
Calories 146, Calories from Fat 0, Total Fat 0 g, Saturated Fat 0 g, Cholesterol 0 mg, Sodium 5 mg, Total Carbohydrate 36 g, Dietary Fiber 5 g, Sugars 28 g, Protein 2 g.

BAKED APPLES WITH POMEGRANATE GLAZE

Makes 6 servings • Serving size: 1 apple with 1/4 cup glaze

Lightly sweetened pomegranate juice thickens while the apples bake, making a luxurious ruby sauce for these cinnamony baked apples.

6 medium Granny Smith or Rome apples (about 2 1/4 pounds)

2 cups pomegranate juice

1/4 cup granulated sugar

2 tablespoons all-purpose flour

2 teaspoons fresh grated orange zest

1/2 teaspoon ground cinnamon

1. Preheat the oven to 350°F. Coat an 11 × 7-inch baking dish with cooking spray and set aside.

2. Core the apples and pare 1 inch of the peel from the tops. Place in the prepared dish. Combine the pomegranate juice, sugar, flour, orange zest, and cinnamon in a medium bowl and whisk until smooth. Pour the pomegranate juice mixture over the apples.

3. Bake, uncovered, 40 to 45 minutes or until the apples are tender, basting twice. Check the apples carefully during the last 10 minutes of baking to prevent overcooking and bursting of the skins. Serve the warm apples in shallow bowls drizzled with the glaze.

Exchanges: 3 Carbohydrate

Calories 178, Calories from Fat 0, Total Fat 0 g, Saturated Fat 0 g, Cholesterol 0 mg, Sodium 5 mg, Total Carbohydrate 46 g, Dietary Fiber 4 g, Sugars 36 g, Protein 1 g.

GINGER POACHED APRICOTS

Makes 6 servings • Serving size: 2 apricot halves with 1 tablespoon syrup

A generous amount of fresh ginger gives these apricots real zing. Cut the amount in half if you prefer a milder flavor. Use the syrup for poaching nectarines or peaches, too.

1/2 cup water

1/4 cup granulated sugar

1/4 cup chopped fresh ginger

2 teaspoons fresh grated lime zest

6 medium apricots (about 3/4 pound), halved and pitted

1. Combine the water, sugar, ginger, and lime zest in a small saucepan and bring to a boil. Reduce the heat to low, cover, and simmer 5 minutes. Cool to room temperature.

2. Strain the sugar mixture through a fine wire mesh sieve into a medium skillet, discarding the solids. Add the apricots to the skillet and bring to a boil. Reduce the heat to low, cover, and simmer until the apricots are tender, 3 to 4 minutes.

3. To serve, spoon the apricots into individual dessert bowls. Drizzle the syrup evenly over the apricots.

Exchanges: 1 Carbohydrate
Calories 61, Calories from Fat 0, Total Fat 0 g, Saturated Fat 0 g, Cholesterol 0 mg, Sodium 1 mg, Total Carbohydrate 15 g, Dietary Fiber 1 g, Sugars 13 g, Protein 1 g.

Maple–Cider Fruit Compote

Makes 8 servings • Serving size: 1/2 cup

Black pepper provides a bit of heat to this spiced compote. Serve it with a
thin slice of plain cake or a simple cookie for an understated dessert.
Or, you can serve it as a sweet side dish with roast pork.

2 cups apple cider

1/4 cup maple syrup

6 whole cloves, crushed

**1 (3-inch) cinnamon stick,
broken into 3 pieces**

**1 (2-inch) piece fresh
ginger, sliced**

**1/2 teaspoon whole
allspice, crushed**

**1/4 teaspoon whole
black peppercorns**

**2 Golden Delicious apples,
peeled, quartered, and cored**

**2 not-too-ripe Bartlett pears,
peeled, quartered, and cored**

1/2 cup dried apricots

1/2 cup dried dates

1/3 cup dried cranberries

1. Combine the cider, maple syrup, cloves, cinnamon, ginger, allspice, and peppercorns in a medium saucepan. Bring to a boil, reduce heat to low, cover, and simmer 15 minutes. Strain and discard the spices.

2. Return the cider mixture to the saucepan. Add the apples, pears, apricots, dates, and cranberries and bring to a boil. Reduce the heat to low and simmer, covered, stirring occasionally, until the pears and apples are just tender, 10 minutes. Let stand to cool to room temperature.

3. The compote may be kept in an airtight container and stored in the refrigerator for up to 3 days. Bring to room temperature before serving.

Exchanges: 3 Fruit

Calories 188, Calories from Fat 0, Total Fat 0 g, Saturated Fat 0 g, Cholesterol 0 mg,
Sodium 6 mg, Total Carbohydrate 49 g, Dietary Fiber 4 g, Sugars 40 g, Protein 1 g.

THREE MELON–MINT COMPOTE

Makes 8 servings • Serving size: 1/2 cup

Marinating this compote overnight infuses the melon with mint flavor. Take it to a summer picnic or a potluck and serve it in a clear bowl to show off all the pretty melon colors.

1 cup water

1/4 cup granulated sugar

1 tablespoon cornstarch

1/4 cup peeled and chopped fresh ginger

1/4 cup plus 2 tablespoons chopped fresh mint, divided use

Pinch of salt

1 1/2 cups 1-inch watermelon balls

1 1/2 cups 1-inch cantaloupe balls

1 cup 1-inch honeydew balls

Fresh mint sprigs (optional)

1. Combine the water, sugar, and cornstarch in a small saucepan and whisk until the cornstarch dissolves. Cook over medium-high heat, 3 to 4 minutes, whisking constantly until the mixture comes to a boil and thickens slightly.

2. Remove from the heat and stir in the ginger, 1/4 cup of the mint, and the salt. Cool to room temperature. Pour the mixture through a fine wire mesh strainer, discarding the solids. Stir in the watermelon, cantaloupe, honeydew, and remaining 2 tablespoons mint.

3. Cover and refrigerate overnight. Spoon into serving bowls and garnish with fresh mint springs, if desired.

Exchanges: 1 Carbohydrate
Calories 58, Calories from Fat 0, Total Fat 0 g, Saturated Fat 0 g, Cholesterol 0 mg, Sodium 26 mg, Total Carbohydrate 14 g, Dietary Fiber 1 g, Sugars 12 g, Protein 1 g.

Sparkling Raspberry–Citrus Fruit Cocktail

Makes 12 servings • Serving size: 1/2 cup

Tart and sweet citrus-flavored raspberry juice makes a delicious base for a fruit cocktail at any time of year. Use whatever fruit is in season—from apples and pears to melon and berries.

3 large navel oranges

1 large lemon

1 lime

1 cup fresh raspberries or unsweetened frozen raspberries, thawed

2 tablespoons superfine sugar

2 cups sliced strawberries

2 cups 1-inch cantaloupe or honeydew balls

4 medium peaches, peeled, pitted, and sliced (about 2 cups)

1/2 cup sparkling water, chilled

1. Combine the zest from two of the oranges, the zest from the lemon and the lime, and the juice from all the oranges, the lemon, and lime in a medium bowl. Add the raspberries and the sugar and crush the berries using a potato masher. Cover and refrigerate overnight.

2. Pour the mixture through a fine wire mesh strainer into a serving bowl, discarding the solids. Add the strawberries, cantaloupe, and peaches. Stir in the sparkling water just before serving.

Exchanges: 1 Fruit

Calories 59, Calories from Fat 0, Total Fat 0 g, Saturated Fat 0 g, Cholesterol 0 mg, Sodium 6 mg, Total Carbohydrate 14 g, Dietary Fiber 2 g, Sugars 12 g, Protein 1 g.

Spiked Peaches with Raspberry Sauce

Makes 8 servings • Serving size: 1/2 cup peaches with 2 tablespoons sauce

Celebrate the all-too-short summer peach season with this easy dessert. Raspberry liqueur "spikes" the peaches, but you can omit it if youngsters are part of the party. The peaches and sauce are delicious on their own, or you can gild the lily with a scoop of fat-free, no-sugar-added vanilla ice cream.

Peaches

4 large ripe peaches (about 1 1/4 pounds), peeled, pitted, and sliced (about 4 cups)

1 tablespoon granulated sugar

1/4 cup raspberry liqueur

Raspberry Sauce

1 (12-ounce) package frozen unsweetened raspberries, thawed

2 tablespoons granulated sugar

1 tablespoon fresh lemon juice

Make Peaches

1. Combine the peaches, sugar, and liqueur in a medium bowl and stir to mix well.

2. Let stand at room temperature for 30 minutes, stirring occasionally.

Make Sauce

1. Combine the raspberries, sugar, and lemon juice in a food processor or blender and puree. Press the mixture through a fine wire mesh sieve, discarding the solids.

2. To serve, spoon about 1/2 cup of the peaches and their juices into each of 8 shallow serving dishes. Drizzle each serving with 2 tablespoons sauce.

Exchanges: 1 Carbohydrate
Calories 78, Calories from Fat 0, Total Fat 0 g, Saturated Fat 0 g, Cholesterol 0 mg, Sodium 1 mg, Total Carbohydrate 16 g, Dietary Fiber 1 g, Sugars 15 g, Protein 1 g.

STRAWBERRY FOOL

Makes 6 servings • Serving size: 1/2 cup Strawberry Fool with 1/4 cup sliced strawberries

A fool is an English dessert, typically made by folding pureed fruit into whipped cream. This lower-fat adaptation is just as good as the original version.

3 1/2 cups sliced strawberries, divided use

1/4 cup granulated sugar

2 cups plain low-fat yogurt

1/2 teaspoon vanilla extract

1. Combine 2 cups of the strawberries and the sugar in a food processor and process until the mixture is pureed.

2. Spoon the yogurt into a medium bowl and stir in the vanilla. Add the pureed strawberry mixture and gently swirl together without mixing completely. Spoon into 6 serving bowls and top evenly with the remaining 1 1/2 cups strawberries.

Exchanges: 1 1/2 Carbohydrate
Calories 110, Calories from Fat 14, Total Fat 2 g, Saturated Fat 1 g, Cholesterol 5 mg, Sodium 54 mg, Total Carbohydrate 20 g, Dietary Fiber 2 g, Sugars 18 g, Protein 5 g,

FRESH BERRY TERRINE

Makes 8 servings • Serving size: 1 (1-inch) slice

If you can boil water, you can make this stunning dessert. Display it on a platter—
no garnish required—and enjoy the compliments. This is definitely a
peak-of-summer dessert—frozen berries just aren't pretty enough.

2 cups light white cranberry juice, divided use

2 envelopes unflavored gelatin

2 cups quartered strawberries

2 cups fresh raspberries

2 cups fresh blueberries

1. Pour 1/2 cup of the cranberry juice into a medium bowl and sprinkle the gelatin over the juice. Let stand 5 minutes to soften.

2. Place 1/2 cup of the remaining cranberry juice in a small saucepan and heat to boiling. Pour over the gelatin mixture and stir until the gelatin dissolves. Stir in the remaining 1 cup cranberry juice.

3. Place the strawberries, raspberries, and blueberries in an 8 × 4-inch loaf pan. Pour the cranberry mixture over the berries. Cover and refrigerate overnight.

4. Run a thin-bladed knife around the edge of the terrine and invert onto a serving platter. Cut into slices using a serrated knife.

Exchanges: 1 Fruit
Calories 63, Calories from Fat 0, Total Fat 0 g, Saturated Fat 0 g, Cholesterol 0 mg, Sodium 23 mg, Total Carbohydrate 14 g, Dietary Fiber 4 g, Sugars 9 g, Protein 2 g.

BLACKBERRIES WITH LIME CREAM

Makes 8 servings • Serving size: 1/2 cup berries with 2 tablespoons Lime Cream

The possibilities for this recipe are almost endless: use any single fruit or
mixture of fruit, and vary the cream by using lemon, orange, or
your favorite liqueur or extract.

1/4 cup cold water

1 tablespoon 100% dried egg
whites or meringue powder

2 tablespoons
granulated sugar

1/3 cup reduced-fat cream
cheese, softened

1/4 cup granular no-calorie
sweetener

2 teaspoons fresh grated
lime zest

2 teaspoons fresh lime juice

1/2 teaspoon vanilla extract

4 cups fresh blackberries

1. Combine water and dried egg whites in a large bowl and
   beat at high speed for 5 minutes or until foamy. Gradually
   beat in the sugar, beating 5 minutes longer or until stiff,
   glossy, and bright white.

2. Combine cream cheese, no-calorie sweetener, lime zest,
   lime juice, and vanilla in a large bowl and stir to mix well.
   Gently fold the egg white mixture into the cream cheese
   mixture in four additions, mixing well after each addition.

3. Spoon the blackberries into 8 serving bowls and spoon
   Lime Cream evenly over the berries.

Exchanges: 1 Carbohydrate
Calories 69, Calories from Fat 10, Total Fat 1 g, Saturated Fat 1 g, Cholesterol 4 mg,
Sodium 18 mg, Total Carbohydrate 14 g, Dietary Fiber 4 g, Sugars 10 g, Protein 2 g

Fruit-Filled Pavlovas with Vanilla Sauce

Makes 6 servings • Serving size: 1 baked meringue with 1/2 cup fruit and 2 tablespoons sauce

Make the baked meringues and the sauce a day ahead for this easy, yet so sophisticated, dessert. Serve it with a single fresh fruit or a colorful mixture of seasonal fruits. To make meringue cookies using the Baked Meringue recipe, make the mounds of egg white mixture about 1 1/2 inches in diameter and bake them for about 40 minutes. Don't make the meringues on a humid day or they will be soggy.

Baked Meringues

2 egg whites

1/4 teaspoon cream of tartar

1 teaspoon vanilla extract

1/4 cup granulated sugar

Vanilla Sauce

1 egg yolk

3/4 cup 1% low-fat milk

3 tablespoons granular no-calorie sweetener

1 teaspoon cornstarch

Pinch of salt

1/2 teaspoon vanilla extract

Filling

3 cups mixed chopped fruit and/or berries

Make Meringues

1. Preheat the oven to 225°F. Line a large baking sheet with parchment paper and set aside.

2. Combine the egg whites and cream of tartar in a medium bowl and beat at medium speed until foamy. Beat in the vanilla. Gradually add the sugar and beat at high speed until stiff peaks form.

3. Place 6 mounds of egg white mixture onto the prepared pan and use the back of a spoon to spread to 3-inch diameter circles, creating indentations in the center of each one. Bake 1 hour or until the meringues are dry. Cool in the pan on a wire rack. Carefully remove the meringues from the paper.

Make Sauce

1. Place the egg yolk in a medium bowl and whisk lightly. Set aside.

2. Combine the milk, no-calorie sweetener, cornstarch, and salt in a medium saucepan and whisk until smooth. Cook over medium heat until bubbles form around the edges of the milk mixture.

3. Slowly whisk about 1/3 cup of the milk mixture into the egg yolk. Whisk the egg yolk mixture into the milk mixture in the saucepan and cook, stirring constantly (do not whisk) until the mixture comes to a boil and thickens. Strain through a fine wire mesh strainer into a medium bowl and cool to room temperature. Stir in the vanilla.

4. To assemble the dessert, place baked meringues on serving plates and top evenly with the fruit. Drizzle each one with 2 tablespoons of the Vanilla Sauce and serve immediately. The meringues can be covered in an airtight container and stored at room temperature up to 1 day. The sauce can be covered and stored refrigerated up to 2 days. Bring to room temperature before serving.

Exchanges: 1 1/2 Carbohydrate
Calories 102, Calories from Fat 13, Total Fat 1 g, Saturated Fat 1 g, Cholesterol 37 mg, Sodium 59 mg, Total Carbohydrate 20 g, Dietary Fiber 2 g, Sugars 17 g, Protein 3 g.

Toasted Almond Napoleon with Berries

Makes 8 servings • Serving size: 1 (1-inch) slice

This show-stopping confection can't be assembled ahead of time—the cake layers get soggy too fast. But, it looks so stunning and tastes so sumptuous it's worth the last-minute effort.

2 cups plain low-fat yogurt

1 1/4 cups slivered almonds

1 tablespoon all-purpose flour

4 egg whites

1/4 teaspoon cream of tartar

1/8 teaspoon salt

1 1/2 teaspoons vanilla extract, divided use

3/4 cup granular no-calorie sweetener, divided use

2 cups fresh raspberries or blueberries

1/2 teaspoon confectioners' sugar

1. Line a sieve or a colander with several thicknesses of cheesecloth or with a coffee filter and set over a bowl. Spoon the yogurt into the sieve, cover, and refrigerate overnight.

2. Preheat the oven to 350°F. Place the almonds in a small baking pan. Bake, stirring once, 8 to 10 minutes or until lightly toasted. Set aside to cool. Maintain the oven temperature.

3. Line the bottom of a 13 × 9-inch baking pan with parchment, leaving a 3-inch overhang of parchment on each 9-inch side of the pan. Coat the parchment and exposed sides of the pan with cooking spray. Set aside.

4. Place the cooled almonds in a food processor and process until finely ground. Place the almonds in a small bowl and stir in the flour. Set aside.

5. Place the egg whites, cream of tartar, and salt in a medium bowl and beat at medium speed until foamy. Beat in 1/2 teaspoon of the vanilla. Slowly beat in 1/2 cup of the no-calorie sweetener and beat at high speed until stiff peaks form.

6. Spoon the almond mixture over the egg white mixture in four additions, mixing until no white streaks remain. Spoon the batter into the prepared pan, spreading evenly. Bake for 10 to 12 minutes or until set. Immediately remove the cake from the pan using the overhanging parchment to lift the cake. Place on a wire rack for 5 minutes to cool slightly. Using the parchment paper, transfer the cake to a cutting board and cut cake into 3 (12 × 3-inch) rectangles with a serrated knife. Discard the parchment paper. Lift each cake rectangle onto a wire rack using a long metal spatula and cool completely.

7. Combine the drained yogurt, remaining 1/4 cup no-calorie sweetener, and remaining 1 teaspoon vanilla in a medium bowl and stir to mix well.

8. To assemble, place one cake rectangle on a serving plate and spread evenly with 1/2 cup of the yogurt mixture. Top with 1 cup of the berries. Repeat layering with the remaining yogurt and berries. Top with the remaining cake rectangle. Sprinkle top of napoleon with confectioners' sugar and serve immediately.

Exchanges: 1 Carbohydrate • 2 1/2 Fat
Calories 189, Calories from Fat 104, Total Fat 12 g, Saturated Fat 1 g, Cholesterol 3 mg, Sodium 99 mg, Total Carbohydrate 14 g, Dietary Fiber 4 g, Sugars 7 g, Protein 9 g.

Custards & Puddings

CHOCOLATE VELVET PUDDING

Makes 4 servings • Serving size: 1/2 cup

The secret to satiny, lump-free pudding is constant whisking while it cooks.
If yours turns out less than perfectly smooth, press the hot pudding
through a fine wire mesh sieve using a rubber spatula.

2 cups fat-free milk

1 large egg

1/3 cup unsweetened cocoa

1/4 cup granulated sugar

1/4 cup granular no-calorie sweetener

3 tablespoons cornstarch

Pinch of salt

2 teaspoons vanilla extract

1. Combine the milk, egg, cocoa, sugar, no-calorie sweetener, cornstarch, and salt in a medium heavy-bottomed saucepan and whisk until cornstarch dissolves. Cook over medium heat, whisking constantly, about 6 minutes or until the mixture comes to a boil and thickens.

2. Transfer to a medium bowl and cover the surface of the pudding with plastic wrap to prevent a skin from forming. Cool to room temperature and stir in the vanilla. Cover and refrigerate 2 hours or until chilled.

Exchanges: 2 Carbohydrate
Calories 162, Calories from Fat 21, Total Fat 2 g, Saturated Fat 1 g, Cholesterol 55 mg, Sodium 121 mg, Total Carbohydrate 30 g, Dietary Fiber 2 g, Sugars 21 g, Protein 7 g.

CLASSIC BANANA PUDDING

Makes 10 servings • Serving size: 1/2 cup

The small amount of sugar in the topping helps the meringue brown to perfection, and a bit of sour cream lends a touch of richness to this wonderful pudding.

3 cups fat-free milk

1 large egg

1/3 cup granular no-calorie sweetener

1/4 cup cornstarch

Pinch of salt

1/3 cup reduced-fat sour cream

2 teaspoons vanilla extract

2 medium ripe bananas, sliced

20 reduced-fat vanilla wafers, divided use

3 egg whites

1/4 teaspoon cream of tartar

1 tablespoon granulated sugar

1. Preheat the oven to 325°F.

2. Combine the milk, egg, no-calorie sweetener, cornstarch, and salt in a medium heavy-bottomed saucepan and whisk until smooth. Cook over medium heat, whisking constantly, about 6 minutes or until the mixture comes to a boil and thickens. Remove from the heat and stir in the sour cream and vanilla.

3. Arrange 1/3 of the banana slices in the bottom of a 1 1/2-quart soufflé or baking dish. Spread 1/3 (about 1 cup) of the custard over the banana. Layer 10 of the wafers on top of the custard. Top with 1/3 of the banana slices and spread another 1/3 of the custard over the bananas. Top with the remaining 10 wafers. Top the wafers with the remaining banana slices and custard.

4. Combine the egg whites and cream of tartar in a large bowl and beat at high speed until foamy. Gradually add the sugar, beating until stiff peaks form. Spread the egg whites evenly over the pudding, sealing to the edge of the dish. Bake for 25 minutes or until the meringue is golden.

5. Cool the pudding to room temperature, then refrigerate at least 2 hours. The pudding is best served within a day of preparation, as the bananas begin to discolor upon standing. Store any leftovers in the refrigerator.

Exchanges: 1 1/2 Carbohydrate • 1/2 Fat
Calories 132, Calories from Fat 21, Total Fat 2 g, Saturated Fat 1 g, Cholesterol 25 mg, Sodium 100 mg, Total Carbohydrate 22 g, Dietary Fiber 1 g, Sugars 13 g, Protein 5g

Apricot–Orange Pudding

Makes 4 servings • Serving size: 1/2 cup pudding with 1/4 cup orange segments

Brighten your day with a bowl of sunny apricot pudding served with sweet orange segments. If you want to chill it quickly, place the bowl of pudding inside a larger bowl of ice water for about 20 minutes and stir occasionally.

2/3 cup fresh-squeezed orange juice	1 large egg
1/3 cup dried apricots, chopped	Pinch of salt
2 cups 1% low-fat milk	1/4 teaspoon almond extract
1/4 cup granulated sugar	2 large navel oranges
3 tablespoons cornstarch	

1. Place the orange juice in a small saucepan and heat over medium heat until hot but not boiling. Remove from heat and add the apricots. Cover and let stand for 15 minutes or until the apricots are very soft. Transfer the apricot mixture to a food processor and process until the apricots are finely chopped. Transfer to a medium bowl.

2. Combine the milk, sugar, cornstarch, egg, and salt in a medium heavy-bottomed saucepan and whisk until the cornstarch dissolves. Cook over medium heat, whisking constantly, about 6 minutes or until the mixture comes to a boil and thickens. Add the milk mixture to the apricot mixture and stir to combine. Cover the surface of the pudding with plastic wrap to prevent a skin from forming. Cool to room temperature and stir in the almond extract. Cover and refrigerate 2 hours or until chilled.

3. Cut a thin slice from the top and bottom of each of the oranges, exposing the flesh. Stand each fruit upright, and using a sharp knife, thickly cut off the peel, following the contour of the fruit and removing all the white pith and membrane. Holding the fruit over a bowl, carefully cut along both sides of each section to free it from the membrane. Discard any seeds and let the sections fall into the bowl.

4. To serve, spoon the pudding into individual dessert bowls. Spoon the orange segments evenly over the pudding.

Exchanges: 3 Carbohydrate • 1/2 Fat
Calories 245, Calories from Fat 25, Total Fat 3 g, Saturated Fat 1 g, Cholesterol 60 mg, Sodium 119 mg, Total Carbohydrate 50 g, Dietary Fiber 3 g, Sugars 40 g, Protein 7 g.

CREAMY RISOTTO PUDDING

Makes 8 servings • Serving size: 1/2 cup

To make this pudding in a slow cooker, combine the milk, rice, brown sugar, and salt in the cooker. Cook on high for 3 1/2 hours, stir in the dried fruit, and cook 30 minutes longer. Add the orange zest and vanilla just before serving.

5 cups 1% low-fat milk

1 cup Arborio or other short grain rice

1/3 cup light brown sugar

1/2 teaspoon salt

1/3 cup dried cherries, cranberries, raisins, currants, or any chopped dried fruit

2 teaspoons fresh grated orange zest

1 teaspoon vanilla extract

1. Combine the milk, rice, brown sugar, and salt in a large saucepan and bring to a boil. Reduce heat to low and simmer, uncovered, stirring often, 12 minutes or until the pudding begins to thicken.

2. Stir in the cherries or other dried fruit and continue cooking and stirring for 8 to 10 minutes or until the rice is tender and most of the milk is absorbed. Stir more frequently as the pudding becomes thicker. Remove from the heat and stir in the orange zest and vanilla.

3. Serve warm or chilled. To chill, cover the surface of the pudding to prevent a skin from forming and refrigerate 4 hours.

Variation

To make Fruited Rice Pudding Brûlée, omit the dried fruit when making the pudding. Place 1/4 cup chopped fresh fruit, such as peaches, nectarines, mangos, or berries, in the bottom of each of 8 custard cups. Top evenly with the warm pudding. Top each serving with 2 teaspoons light brown sugar. Place the custard cups in a baking pan. Broil 2 inches from heat source until the sugar is completely melted and caramelized.

Exchanges: 2 1/2 Carbohydrate
Calories 197, Calories from Fat 15, Total Fat 2 g, Saturated Fat 1 g, Cholesterol 9 mg, Sodium 228 mg, Total Carbohydrate 38 g, Dietary Fiber 0 g, Sugars 19 g, Protein 7 g.

Mango Swirl Tapioca Pudding

Makes 4 servings • Serving size: 1/2 cup

Fresh fruit puree and exotic cardamom liven up a childhood classic. Substitute fresh or frozen peaches for the mango if you wish. Make these into tapioca mango parfaits by layering cubes of fresh mango alternately with the pudding into tall glasses.

2 cups fat-free milk

1 large egg

1/3 cup granulated sugar

3 tablespoons minute tapioca

1/4 teaspoon salt

1/8 teaspoon ground cardamom

1 teaspoon vanilla extract

1 medium ripe mango, peeled, pitted, and chopped

1. Combine the milk, egg, sugar, tapioca, salt, and cardamom in a medium heavy-bottomed saucepan, stirring to mix well. Let stand for 5 minutes.

2. Cook the milk mixture over medium heat, stirring constantly, about 6 minutes or until the mixture comes to a full boil. Transfer to a medium bowl and cover the surface of the pudding with plastic wrap to prevent a skin from forming. Cool to room temperature. Stir in the vanilla, cover, and refrigerate 2 hours or until chilled.

3. Place the mango in a food processor and process until smooth. (You should have about 1/2 cup mango puree). Gently fold the mango puree into the pudding, creating a swirled effect.

Exchanges: 2 1/2 Carbohydrate
Calories 195, Calories from Fat 14, Total Fat 2 g, Saturated Fat 1 g, Cholesterol 55 mg, Sodium 229 mg, Total Carbohydrate 40 g, Dietary Fiber 1 g, Sugars 31 g, Protein 6 g.

Silky Baked Egg Custards

Makes 4 servings • Serving size: 1 baked custard

Serve these yummy egg custards, lightly speckled with nutmeg, with a few vanilla wafers alongside or topped with fresh, colorful berries. Because the custards continue to cook if left in the water bath, carefully lift them out with a metal spatula as soon as they are done.

1 large egg

1 egg white

1/3 cup granulated sugar

1/8 teaspoon ground nutmeg

1 1/2 cups 1% low-fat milk

1 teaspoon vanilla extract

1. Preheat the oven to 325°F.

2. Combine the egg, egg white, sugar, and nutmeg in a medium bowl. Whisk until smooth and set aside.

3. Heat the milk over medium-high heat in a small saucepan until bubbles form around the edges. (Do not allow to come to a boil.) Slowly whisk the hot milk into the egg mixture. Whisk in the vanilla. Divide the mixture evenly among 6 (6-ounce) custard cups. Place the cups inside a baking pan and add hot water to level halfway up the cups.

4. Bake for 45 to 50 minutes or until almost set but still a bit soft in the center. The custards should wiggle a bit when you shake the cups, but will firm up as they cool. Remove the custards from the water bath and let cool to room temperature. Serve at room temperature or chilled.

Exchanges: 1 1/2 Carbohydrate • 1/2 Fat
Calories 131, Calories from Fat 20, Total Fat 2 g, Saturated Fat 1 g, Cholesterol 59 mg, Sodium 78 mg, Total Carbohydrate 22 g, Dietary Fiber 0 g, Sugars 21 g, Protein 5 g.

Cappuccino Crème Brûlée

Makes 8 servings • Serving size: 1 crème brûlée

The coffee flavor in these custards is delicate—it's more of a gentle nudge than a jolt. If you love a bold coffee taste, simply increase the amount of espresso or coffee granules. The creamy cappuccino custard and the sweet brown sugar topping combine perfectly in this luxurious and impressive dessert.

2 large eggs

2 egg whites

1/3 cup granulated sugar

1/3 cup granular no-calorie sweetener

3 cups 1% low-fat milk

1 1/2 teaspoons espresso granules or 1 tablespoon instant coffee granules

1 teaspoon vanilla extract

16 teaspoons light brown sugar

1. Preheat the oven to 325°F.
2. Combine the eggs, egg whites, sugar, and no-calorie sweetener in a medium bowl and whisk until smooth. Set aside.
3. Combine the milk and espresso granules in a small saucepan. Cook over medium-high heat until bubbles form around the edges. (Do not allow to come to a boil.) Slowly whisk the hot milk into the egg mixture. Whisk in the vanilla. Divide the mixture evenly among 8 (6-ounce) crème brûlée cups or custard cups. Place the cups inside a baking pan and add water to the baking pan to a level halfway up cups.
4. Bake 40 to 45 minutes or until custards are almost set but still a bit soft in the centers. The custards should wiggle a bit when you shake the cups, but will firm up as they cool. Remove the custards from the water bath, let stand just until cool to the touch, and cover the surface of the custards with plastic wrap to prevent a film from forming. Refrigerate 4 hours.
5. Preheat the broiler. Place the custards in a baking pan and top each one with 2 teaspoons of the brown sugar. Broil the custards 2 to 3 minutes until the sugar melts and caramelizes, rearranging the cups as needed for even browning. Remove the individual custards as they are ready. Let the custards stand 5 minutes before serving.

Exchanges: 1 1/2 Carbohydrate • 1/2 Fat
Calories 136, Calories from Fat 20, Total Fat 2 g, Saturated Fat 1 g, Cholesterol 59 mg, Sodium 82 mg, Total Carbohydrate 23 g, Dietary Fiber 0 g, Sugars 23 g, Protein 5 g.

LIVELY LEMON MOUSSE

Makes 8 servings • Serving size: 1/2 cup

Serve this puckery mousse with fresh berries for a tart–sweet springtime dessert. It's a refreshing finish to a celebration meal of lamb or ham. Garnish each serving with strips of lemon zest and fresh strawberries or raspberries.

1/2 cup plain low-fat yogurt

2 teaspoons fresh grated lemon zest

2 tablespoons plus 1/4 cup fresh lemon juice, divided use

1 envelope unflavored gelatin

4 egg whites

1/2 cup granulated sugar

1. Combine the yogurt and lemon zest in a medium bowl and stir to mix well. Set aside.

2. Place 2 tablespoons of the lemon juice in a small saucepan, sprinkle with the gelatin, and let stand to soften for 1 minute. Cook over low heat, stirring constantly for 1 minute or until the gelatin dissolves. Cool slightly. (Don't do this step too far in advance. The mixture must be liquid when it is added to the egg whites.)

3. Combine the egg whites, sugar, and remaining 1/4 cup lemon juice in the top of a double boiler. Place over simmering (not boiling) water and beat at high speed until soft peaks form (about 5 minutes).

4. Remove from the heat and beat in the gelatin mixture. Gently stir about 1/2 cup of the egg white mixture into the yogurt mixture. Fold in the remaining egg white mixture in two additions, mixing until no white streaks remain. Cover and refrigerate 2 hours or until set.

Exchanges: 1 Carbohydrate
Calories 71, Calories from Fat 0, Total Fat 0 g, Saturated Fat 0 g, Cholesterol 1 mg, Sodium 41 mg, Total Carbohydrate 15 g, Dietary Fiber 0 g, Sugars 14 g, Protein 3 g.

CHOCOLATE MOUSSE

Makes 5 servings • Serving size: 1/2 cup

Ethereally light and nearly fat-free, you can enjoy this rich chocolaty treat anytime. It's best served within a day of making because the mousse begins to lose volume after a longer time in the refrigerator.

1/3 cup unsweetened cocoa

1/4 cup boiling water

1/2 cup granulated sugar

4 egg whites

2 tablespoons cool water

1/4 teaspoon cream of tartar

1. Place the cocoa in a medium bowl and pour in 1/4 cup boiling water, stirring until the mixture is smooth.

2. Combine the sugar, egg whites, 2 tablespoons cool water, and the cream of tartar in the top of a double boiler. Place over simmering (not boiling) water and beat at high speed until soft peaks form, about 5 minutes.

3. Remove from the heat and gently stir about 1/2 cup of egg white mixture into the chocolate mixture. Gently fold in the remaining egg white mixture in two additions, mixing until no white streaks remain. Cover and refrigerate 2 hours or until chilled.

Exchanges: 1 1/2 Carbohydrate
Calories 104, Calories from Fat 7, Total Fat 1 g, Saturated Fat 1 g, Cholesterol 0 mg, Sodium 45 mg, Total Carbohydrate 23 g, Dietary Fiber 2 g, Sugars 21 g, Protein 4 g.

PUMPKIN FLAN

Makes 8 servings • Serving size: 1 slice

This silky flan tastes like an ultra-creamy pumpkin pie—without the crust.
Serve it on a rimmed serving plate to avoid spilling any of the delectable caramel syrup.
Make the caramel in a light-colored saucepan so you will be able
to see when the sugar has turned a golden color.

1/2 cup granulated sugar

2 tablespoons water

1 (15-ounce) can 100% pure pumpkin
(not pumpkin pie filling)

1 (12-ounce) can fat-free evaporated milk

1/2 cup light brown sugar

2 tablespoons canola oil

2 large eggs, lightly beaten

1 teaspoon vanilla extract

1/2 teaspoon ground cinnamon

1/4 teaspoon ground allspice

1/4 teaspoon ground cloves

1/4 teaspoon salt

1. Preheat the oven to 350°F.

2. Coat the inside rim of a 9-inch round cake pan with cooking spray. Wipe away any cooking spray on the bottom of the pan with a paper towel and set the pan aside.

3. Stir together the sugar and water in a small heavy-bottomed saucepan. Cook over medium heat, stirring constantly, about 3 minutes or until sugar dissolves. Continue cooking without stirring about 4 minutes or until mixture is golden. Carefully pour into the prepared pan, tilting the pan to coat the bottom. The mixture will be very hot. Do not touch the bottom of the pan after pouring in the caramel.

4. Combine the pumpkin, evaporated milk, brown sugar, oil, eggs, vanilla, cinnamon, allspice, cloves, and salt in a large bowl and whisk until the mixture is smooth. Pour over the caramel in the pan. Place the baking pan inside a roasting pan and add hot water to a level halfway up the pan.

5. Bake 35 to 40 minutes or until a knife inserted in the edge of the flan comes out clean and the flan is still a bit soft in the center. The flan should wiggle a bit when you shake the pan, but it will firm up as it cools. Remove the flan from the water bath and cool in the pan on a wire rack 30 minutes. Cover and refrigerate overnight. Loosen the flan by running a small spatula around the edge. Carefully invert the flan onto a rimmed serving plate to avoid spilling the syrup.

Exchanges: 2 1/2 Carbohydrate • 1/2 Fat
Calories 207, Calories from Fat 45, Total Fat 5 g, Saturated Fat 1 g, Cholesterol 55 mg, Sodium 154 mg, Total Carbohydrate 36 g, Dietary Fiber 2 g, Sugars 33 g, Protein 6 g.

MAPLE–GINGER POTS DE CRÈME

Makes 6 servings • Serving size: 1 pot de crème

A sophisticated version of baked custard, this grown-up pudding stays soft in the center with a silky texture and delicate ginger flavor. Don't use substitutes for the maple syrup. It lends an earthy undertone of unique flavor, and with only 24 grams of carb in a serving of this pudding, there's no reason not to use the real thing!

2 large eggs

2 egg whites

1/2 cup maple syrup

1/4 teaspoon fresh grated ginger

Pinch of salt

2 1/2 cups 1% low-fat milk

1. Combine the eggs, egg whites, maple syrup, ginger, and salt in a medium bowl, whisk until smooth, and set aside.

2. Heat the milk over medium-high heat in a small saucepan until bubbles form around the edges. (Do not allow to boil). Slowly whisk the hot milk into the maple syrup mixture. Divide the mixture evenly among 6 (6-ounce) pot de crème cups or custard cups. Place the cups inside a baking pan and add hot water to the baking pan to a level halfway up cups.

3. Bake 45 to 50 minutes or until custards are almost set but still a bit soft in the centers. The custards should wiggle a bit when you shake the cups, but will firm up as they cool. Remove the custards from the water bath, let stand until just cool to the touch, and cover the surface of the cups with plastic wrap to prevent skins from forming. Refrigerate 4 hours.

Exchanges: 1 1/2 Carbohydrate • 1/2 Fat
Calories 145, Calories from Fat 25, Total Fat 3 g, Saturated Fat 1 g, Cholesterol 77 mg, Sodium 120 mg, Total Carbohydrate 24 g, Dietary Fiber 0 g, Sugars 21 g, Protein 7 g.

Buttermilk Panna Cotta with Crushed Raspberries

Makes 6 servings • Serving size: 1 panna cotta with 2 1/2 tablespoons raspberries

The tang of this velvety custard plays off the sweetness of the berries. Make it in summer with fresh raspberries and in winter with the frozen variety.

1 cup 1% low-fat milk

1 1/2 teaspoons unflavored gelatin

1/3 cup granulated sugar

Pinch of salt

1 1/2 cups low-fat buttermilk

1 (12-ounce) package unsweetened frozen raspberries, thawed

1 tablespoon superfine sugar

1. Place the milk in a medium saucepan and sprinkle the gelatin over the milk. Let stand 2 minutes to soften. Add the sugar and salt and cook the mixture over medium heat, stirring often, about 2 minutes or until the sugar dissolves. Remove from heat and stir in the buttermilk. Divide the mixture among 6 (4-ounce) ramekins and refrigerate 4 hours or until set.

2. About an hour before serving, place the berries in a large shallow dish. Add the superfine sugar and stir to combine. Let stand at room temperature, stirring occasionally. Using a fork, lightly crush the berries.

3. To serve, loosen the edges of each panna cotta with the tip of a knife and invert the ramekins onto individual plates. Top each one evenly with the crushed raspberries.

Exchanges: 1 1/2 Carbohydrate
Calories 116, Calories from Fat 9, Total Fat 1 g, Saturated Fat 1 g, Cholesterol 5 mg, Sodium 87 mg, Total Carbohydrate 47 g, Dietary Fiber 0 g, Sugars 23 g, Protein 4 g.

Peach Ladyfinger Trifle

Makes 10 servings • Serving size: 1/2 cup pudding and fruit mixture and 2 ladyfinger halves

Served in a clear glass trifle bowl, this layered dessert makes a lovely presentation. Savor the delicate and comforting combination of pudding and fruit on a midsummer night when peaches are at their flavorful best.

4 large ripe but firm peaches (about 1 1/4 pounds), peeled, pitted, and sliced (about 4 cups)

1 1/4 cups peach nectar, divided use

2 cups 1% low-fat milk

1 large egg

1/3 cup granulated sugar

1/3 cup granular no-calorie sweetener

1/4 cup cornstarch

Pinch of salt

1/4 cup reduced-fat sour cream

1/2 teaspoon almond extract

10 purchased ladyfingers

1. Combine the peaches and 1 cup of the peach nectar in a medium skillet and bring to a boil. Reduce heat to low, cover, and simmer 3 minutes or until peaches are soft but still maintain their shape. Drain, reserving the cooking liquid.

2. Combine the reserved peach cooking liquid, milk, egg, sugar, no-calorie sweetener, cornstarch, and salt in a medium heavy-bottomed saucepan and whisk until the cornstarch dissolves. Cook over medium heat, whisking constantly, about 6 minutes or until mixture comes to a boil and thickens. Remove from the heat and stir in the sour cream. Transfer to a medium bowl and cover the surface of the pudding with plastic wrap to prevent a skin from forming. Cool to room temperature and stir in the almond extract.

3. Cut the ladyfingers to extend about 1/2-inch from the top of a 1 1/2-quart trifle bowl or soufflé dish when positioned upright from the bottom of the bowl. Split the ladyfingers in half lengthwise using a serrated knife. Brush the cut side of the ladyfingers with the remaining 1/4 cup peach nectar.

4. Spoon 1 cup of the pudding into trifle bowl. Line the side of the bowl with ladyfingers, positioning upright with cut sides facing inward. Reserve 5 peach slices for the top of the trifle. Layer the remaining pudding and peach slices into the trifle bowl, ending with pudding. Arrange the reserved peach slices on top of the pudding in a pinwheel design. Serve immediately or cover and refrigerate overnight (the ladyfingers will soften).

Exchanges: 2 Carbohydrate
Calories 141, Calories from Fat 17, Total Fat 2 g, Saturated Fat 1 g, Cholesterol 32 mg, Sodium 62 mg, Total Carbohydrate 28 g, Dietary Fiber 1 g, Sugars 20 g, Protein 4 g.

AMBROSIA TRIFLE

Makes 20 servings • Serving size: 1/2 cup

When you need to serve a crowd for a potluck or a holiday get-together, choose this stunning fruit and cake dessert. Usually made with heavy cream and lots of nuts, this low-fat trifle has a light orange custard, lots of fruit, and a garnish of coconut.

Cake

2 cups cake flour

2 teaspoons baking powder

1 teaspoon baking soda

1/4 teaspoon salt

1/4 cup canola oil

1 large egg

1/3 cup granulated sugar

1/3 cup granular no-calorie sweetener

1 1/3 cups low-fat buttermilk

1 tablespoon vanilla extract

1 tablespoon fresh grated orange zest

Custard

1 cup fat-free milk

1 (6-ounce) container frozen orange juice concentrate, thawed

1/3 cup granular no-calorie sweetener

3 tablespoons cornstarch

1/4 teaspoon salt

1/4 cup reduced-fat sour cream

1 tablespoon fresh grated orange zest

Fruit

4 large oranges

2 cups sliced fresh strawberries

1 medium banana, sliced

Garnish

2 tablespoons sweetened flaked coconut, toasted

Make Cake

1. Preheat the oven to 350°F. Coat a 13 × 9-inch baking pan with cooking spray and set aside.

2. Combine the flour, baking powder, baking soda, and salt in a medium bowl and whisk to mix well.

3. Combine the oil and egg in a large bowl and beat at medium speed until well mixed. Gradually add the sugar and no-calorie sweetener and beat until the mixture is smooth. Add the flour mixture and the buttermilk alternately to the oil mixture, beginning and ending with the flour mixture, beating well after each addition. Beat in the vanilla and stir in the orange zest.

4. Spoon the batter into the prepared pan, smooth the top, and bake for 12 to 15 minutes or until a wooden toothpick inserted in the center of the cake comes out clean. Cool the cake in the pan on a wire rack for 10 minutes. Remove from the pan and cool completely on the wire rack. Cut the cake into 1-inch cubes.

Make Custard

1. Combine the milk, orange juice concentrate, no-calorie sweetener, cornstarch and salt in a medium heavy-bottomed saucepan and whisk until the cornstarch dissolves. Cook over medium heat, whisking constantly, about 6 minutes or until the mixture comes to a boil and thickens.

2. Remove from the heat and whisk in the sour cream. Stir in the orange zest. Transfer to a medium bowl and cover the surface of the custard with plastic wrap to prevent a skin from forming. Cool to room temperature.

Assemble Trifle

1. Cut a thin slice from the top and bottom of each of the oranges, exposing the flesh. Stand each fruit upright, and using a sharp knife, thickly cut off the peel, following the contour of the fruit and removing all the white pith and membrane. Holding the fruit over a bowl, carefully cut along both sides of each section to free it from the membrane. Discard any seeds and let the sections fall into the bowl.

2. Arrange 1/3 of the cake cubes in a 4-quart trifle bowl, top with 1/3 of the custard, 1/3 of the oranges, 1/3 of the strawberries, and 1/3 of the banana slices. Repeat the layering twice with the remaining ingredients. Sprinkle the trifle with coconut just before serving.

Exchanges: 2 Carbohydrate • 1/2 Fat
Calories 162, Calories from Fat 34, Total Fat 4 g, Saturated Fat 1 g, Cholesterol 13 mg, Sodium 189 mg, Total Carbohydrate 29 g, Dietary Fiber 2 g, Sugars 15 g, Protein 3 g.

Rum Raisin Tiramisu

Makes 8 servings • Serving size: 1 slice

When the occasion calls for a sophisticated dessert, make this fabulous rum-soaked layer cake, filled with a delicious raisin-studded custard and topped with chocolate.

Cake

1 cup cake flour

1 teaspoon baking powder

1/2 teaspoon baking soda

Pinch of salt

2 tablespoons canola oil

1 large egg

1/4 cup granular no-calorie sweetener

3 tablespoons granulated sugar

3/4 cup low-fat buttermilk

1 teaspoon vanilla extract

Filling

1 1/2 cups fat-free milk

1 large egg

1/2 cup granular no-calorie sweetener

2 tablespoons cornstarch

Pinch of salt

3 tablespoons reduced-fat cream cheese

1/4 cup raisins

2 tablespoons rum

Topping

1/4 cup brewed espresso or strong coffee, cooled

1 tablespoon rum

1 teaspoon unsweetened cocoa

Make Cake

1. Preheat the oven to 350°F. Coat a 9 × 5-inch loaf pan with cooking spray and set aside.

2. Combine the flour, baking powder, baking soda, and salt in a medium bowl and whisk to mix well. Set aside.

3. Combine the oil and egg in a large bowl and beat at medium speed until well mixed. Gradually add the no-calorie sweetener and sugar and beat until mixture is smooth. Reduce the speed to low and add the flour mixture and the buttermilk alternately to the oil mixture, beginning and ending with the flour mixture, beating well after each addition. Beat in the vanilla.

4. Spoon the batter into the prepared pan and bake for 20 minutes or until a wooden toothpick inserted in the center of the cake comes out clean. Cool the cake in the pan on a wire rack for 10 minutes. Remove from the pan and cool completely on the wire rack.

Make Filling

1. Combine the milk, egg, no-calorie sweetener, cornstarch, and salt in a medium heavy-bottomed saucepan and whisk until smooth. Cook over medium heat, whisking constantly, about 6 minutes or until the mixture comes to a boil and thickens. Remove from the heat and add the cream cheese, whisking until smooth. Stir in the raisins and rum.

2. Transfer to a medium bowl and cover the surface of the filling with plastic wrap to prevent a skin from forming. Cool completely.

Assemble Tiramisu

1. Line a 9 × 5-inch loaf pan with plastic wrap, leaving a 4-inch overhang on each side.

2. Combine the espresso and rum in a small bowl.

3. Cut the cooled cake horizontally into 3 layers using a serrated knife. Brush the cut side of the bottom and top layers and one side of the center layer with espresso mixture. Place the bottom layer of the cake in the prepared pan and top with half of the filling. Place the center cake layer over the filling. Top with the remainder of the filling. Place the top layer of the cake over the filling.

4. Cover and refrigerate overnight. Lift the cake from the pan using the overhanging sides of the plastic wrap and sprinkle the top of the cake with cocoa. Carefully transfer the cake to a serving plate.

Exchanges: 2 Carbohydrate • 1 Fat
Calories 207, Calories from Fat 51, Total Fat 6 g, Saturated Fat 1 g, Cholesterol 57 mg, Sodium 232 mg, Total Carbohydrate 30 g, Dietary Fiber 1 g, Sugars 14 g, Protein 6 g.

CARAMEL APPLE BREAD PUDDING

Makes 10 servings • Serving size: 1/2 cup

Caramelizing the apples with brown sugar intensifies the flavor of this nourishing dessert. For variety, substitute raisins or dried cranberries for the currants and fresh pears instead of apples.

2 teaspoons canola oil

3 medium Granny Smith apples (about 1 1/4 pounds), peeled, cored, and cut into 1/2-inch cubes (about 3 1/2 cups)

1 tablespoon plus 1/4 cup light brown sugar, divided use

2 cups 1% low-fat milk

1 large egg

1 egg white

1 teaspoon vanilla extract

1/4 cup granular no-calorie sweetener

1/2 teaspoon ground cinnamon

1/4 teaspoon ground nutmeg

1/8 teaspoon salt

6 slices 100% whole-wheat sandwich bread, toasted, crusts trimmed, and cut into 1/2-inch pieces (about 5 cups)

2 tablespoons dried currants

1. Heat the oil in a large nonstick skillet over medium heat. Add the apples and cook, stirring occasionally, 4 minutes or until apples begin to soften. Stir in 1 tablespoon of the brown sugar and cook, stirring occasionally, about 4 minutes longer or until the apples are lightly browned. Apples should be tender but retain their shape.

2. Combine the milk, egg, egg white, vanilla, no-calorie sweetener, remaining 1/4 cup brown sugar, cinnamon, nutmeg, and salt in a large bowl and whisk until smooth. Add the bread and currants and stir to combine. Gently stir in the apples. Let the mixture stand for 30 minutes, stirring occasionally, until almost all the liquid is absorbed.

3. Preheat the oven to 350°F. Coat an 8-inch round cake pan with cooking spray and spoon the bread mixture into the prepared pan. Place the cake pan in a large baking pan and add hot water to the baking pan to reach a level halfway up the cake pan.

4. Bake until the top of the bread pudding is golden and the pudding is set, about 50 minutes. Let stand 10 minutes before serving. Serve warm.

Exchanges: 1 1/2 Carbohydrate • 1/2 Fat
Calories 137, Calories from Fat 24, Total Fat 3 g, Saturated Fat 1 g, Cholesterol 24 mg, Sodium 144 mg, Total Carbohydrate 25 g, Dietary Fiber 2 g, Sugars 18 g, Protein 4 g.

BLUEBERRY–NECTARINE CLAFOUTI

Makes 8 servings • Serving size: 1 slice

Clafouti is a simple French dessert made by topping fruits or berries with a sweetened batter.
Try baking it with peaches, apricots, or plums instead of nectarines—
and experiment with blackberries, raspberries, or cherries instead of blueberries.

4 medium nectarines (about 1 pound), peeled, pitted, and sliced (about 3 cups)

1 cup fresh blueberries

3/4 cup all-purpose flour

1/3 cup granulated sugar

1/4 cup granular no-calorie sweetener

1 teaspoon baking powder

1/2 teaspoon baking soda

1/4 teaspoon salt

3/4 cup low-fat buttermilk

1/4 cup reduced-fat sour cream

1 large egg

1 teaspoon vanilla extract

1. Preheat the oven to 350°F. Coat a 9 1/2–inch deep-dish glass pie plate with cooking spray. Place the nectarines and blueberries in the prepared pie plate.

2. Combine the flour, sugar, no-calorie sweetener, baking powder, baking soda, salt, buttermilk, sour cream, egg, and vanilla in a large bowl and whisk until smooth. Pour the batter evenly over the fruit.

3. Bake 25 to 30 minutes or until the top is lightly browned. Cool on a rack for 10 minutes before serving. Serve warm.

Exchanges: 2 Carbohydrate
Calories 149, Calories from Fat 17, Total Fat 2 g, Saturated Fat 1 g, Cholesterol 30 mg, Sodium 236 mg, Total Carbohydrate 30 g, Dietary Fiber 2 g, Sugars 18 g, Protein 4 g.

RASPBERRY–LEMON PUDDING CAKE

Makes 8 servings • Serving size: 1/2 cup

Pudding cakes have just a handful of flour, giving them a light texture and a soufflé-like center. Don't expect to serve this cake in neat slices—it's a spoonable serve-in-a-bowl kind of dessert. The sweet berries play off the tangy lemon cake, making a delightful finish for a summer lunch.

1/2 cup granulated sugar

1/4 cup all-purpose flour

Pinch of salt

1/2 cup plain low-fat yogurt

1/2 cup 1% low-fat milk

2 teaspoons fresh grated lemon zest

1/4 cup fresh lemon juice

2 tablespoons canola oil

1 egg yolk

2 egg whites

1 cup fresh raspberries

1/2 teaspoon confectioners' sugar

1. Preheat the oven to 350°F. Coat a 9-inch round cake pan with cooking spray and set aside.

2. Combine the granulated sugar, flour, salt, yogurt, milk, lemon zest, lemon juice, oil, and egg yolk in a medium bowl and whisk until the mixture is smooth.

3. Place the egg whites in a medium bowl and beat at high speed until soft peaks form. Gently fold 1/4 of the egg white mixture into the sugar mixture. Gently fold in the remaining egg white mixture in two additions, mixing until no white streaks remain. Fold in the raspberries. Spoon the batter into prepared pan.

4. Place the cake pan in a large baking pan and add hot water to the baking pan to a level halfway up cake pan. Bake 35 minutes or until the cake springs back when touched in the center and tiny cracks appear on the surface. (The cake will not be browned.) Sprinkle the top of the cake with confectioners' sugar and serve warm from the pan.

Exchanges: 1 1/2 Carbohydrate • 1/2 Fat
Calories 131, Calories from Fat 42, Total Fat 5 g, Saturated Fat 1 g, Cholesterol 28 mg, Sodium 52 mg, Total Carbohydrate 20 g, Dietary Fiber 1 g, Sugars 15 g, Protein 3 g.

Strawberries with Orange Zabaglione

Makes 6 servings • Serving size: 1/2 cup berries with 1/2 cup sauce

Whether spooned over fresh berries or a simple slice of cake, this frothy custard turns any dessert into a pure delight. Make it with almost any liqueur—try Frangelico, Chambord, Amaretto, or Crème de Cassis. Make sure whatever you choose to serve it with is ready before you begin to make the custard—you'll need to pour it directly from the pan over the berries or cake.

3 cups sliced fresh strawberries

1/4 cup granulated sugar

4 egg yolks

1/4 cup orange or other flavored liqueur

1. Divide the strawberries evenly among six stemmed glasses or small bowls.

2. Combine the sugar and egg yolks in the top of a double boiler and whisk until smooth. Whisk in the liqueur and place the top of the double boiler over barely simmering (not boiling) water. Beat the mixture at high speed for about 6 minutes or until soft peaks form.

3. Spoon the sauce over the berries and serve immediately.

Exchanges: 1 1/2 Carbohydrate • 1/2 Fat
Calories 135, Calories from Fat 34, Total Fat 4 g, Saturated Fat 1 g, Cholesterol 142 mg, Sodium 7 mg, Total Carbohydrate 20 g, Dietary Fiber 2 g, Sugars 18 g, Protein 2g.

Cookies & Bars

CHEWY CHOCOLATE CHIP COOKIES

Makes 25 servings • Serving size: 2 (1 1/2-inch) cookies

These chubby cookies are moist and chewy. If you like yours thin and crisp,
substitute 1 cup of granulated sugar for the 3/4 cup brown sugar and
drop the mounds of dough about 2 inches apart.

1 1/2 cups all-purpose flour

1/4 teaspoon salt

1/4 teaspoon baking soda

1/4 cup 67% vegetable oil butter-flavored spread, at room temperature

3/4 cup light brown sugar

1 large egg

2 teaspoons vanilla extract

2/3 cup miniature chocolate chips

1. Preheat the oven to 350°F. Line baking sheets with parchment paper and set aside.

2. Combine the flour, salt, and baking soda in a medium bowl and whisk to mix well. Set aside.

3. Combine the butter-flavored spread and brown sugar in a large bowl and beat at medium speed until the mixture is well combined. Beat in the egg and vanilla. Add the flour mixture and beat at low speed until thoroughly combined. Stir in the chocolate chips.

4. Drop mounds of dough, about 2 teaspoons each, 1 inch apart, onto prepared baking sheets. Bake 12 minutes or until the bottoms of the cookies are lightly browned.

5. Cool the cookies on the baking sheets on wire racks for 2 minutes. Remove from the baking sheets and cool completely on the wire racks. The cookies can be covered in an airtight container and stored at room temperature up to 2 days.

Exchanges: 1 Carbohydrate • 1/2 Fat
Calories 90, Calories from Fat 25, Total Fat 3 g, Saturated Fat 1 g, Cholesterol 10 mg, Sodium 55 mg, Total Carbohydrate 15 g, Dietary Fiber 0 g, Sugars 9 g, Protein 1 g.

OATMEAL CHOCOLATE CHIPPERS

Makes 15 servings • Serving size: 2 (2-inch) cookies

Kids will hurry off the school bus if they know you've got these crispy chocolate-and-nut-packed cookies waiting for them. Quick to make with ordinary ingredients from the pantry, this recipe is sure to become a family standby.

1/4 cup chopped pecans

1 cup old-fashioned (not quick-cooking) oats

1/4 cup all-purpose flour

1/4 cup whole wheat flour

1/2 teaspoon ground cinnamon

1/4 teaspoon baking soda

1/4 teaspoon salt

1/4 cup natural creamy peanut butter

2 tablespoons 67% vegetable oil butter-flavored spread, at room temperature

1/2 cup light brown sugar

1/4 cup granulated sugar

1 large egg

2 teaspoons vanilla extract

1/4 cup miniature chocolate chips

1. Preheat the oven to 350°F. Place the pecans in a small baking pan and bake until lightly toasted, 5 to 6 minutes. Maintain the oven temperature. Set the pecans aside to cool.

2. Line baking sheets with parchment paper and set aside.

3. Combine the oats, all-purpose flour, whole wheat flour, cinnamon, baking soda, and salt in a medium bowl and whisk to mix well. Set aside.

4. Combine the peanut butter and butter-flavored spread in a large mixing bowl and beat at medium speed until the mixture is fluffy. Add the brown sugar and granulated sugar and beat until well combined. Beat in the egg and vanilla. Add the oat mixture and beat at low speed until moistened. Stir in the chocolate chips and pecans.

5. Drop mounds of dough, 1 level tablespoon each, 2 inches apart, on the prepared baking sheets. Bake until the bottoms of the cookies are lightly browned but the centers remain soft, 10 to 12 minutes.

6. Cool the cookies on the baking sheets on wire racks for 5 minutes. Remove from the baking sheets and cool completely on the wire racks. The cookies can be covered in an airtight container and stored at room temperature up to 2 days.

Exchanges: 1 1/2 Carbohydrate • 1 Fat
Calories 145, Calories from Fat 55, Total Fat 6 g, Saturated Fat 1 g, Cholesterol 15 mg, Sodium 95 mg, Total Carbohydrate 20 g, Dietary Fiber 1 g, Sugars 13 g, Protein 3 g.

CRISPY OATMEAL–RAISIN COOKIES

Makes 22 servings • Serving size: 2 (1 1/2-inch) cookies

These are a crispy, chompy version of the American classic. Filled with hearty whole wheat flour, oats, and just enough sugar, they're a treat you don't have to feel guilty about.

1 1/2 cups old-fashioned (not quick-cooking) oats

1/2 cup all-purpose flour

1/2 cup whole wheat flour

2 teaspoons ground cinnamon

1/2 teaspoon baking soda

1/4 teaspoon salt

1/3 cup 67% vegetable oil butter-flavored spread, at room temperature

1/2 cup dark brown sugar

1/4 cup granulated sugar

1 large egg

1 teaspoon vanilla extract

1/4 cup raisins

1. Preheat the oven to 350°F. Line baking sheets with parchment paper and set aside.

2. Combine the oats, all-purpose flour, whole wheat flour, cinnamon, baking soda, and salt in a medium bowl and whisk to mix well. Set aside.

3. Combine the butter-flavored spread, brown sugar, and granulated sugar in a large mixing bowl and beat at medium speed until the mixture is fluffy. Beat in the egg and vanilla. Add the oat mixture and beat at low speed until moistened. Stir in the raisins.

4. Drop mounds of dough, 2 level teaspoons each, 2 inches apart, on the prepared baking sheets. Bake until the bottoms of the cookies are lightly browned but the centers remain soft, 10 to 12 minutes.

5. Cool the cookies on the baking sheets on wire racks for 2 minutes. Remove from the baking sheets and cool completely on the wire racks. The cookies can be covered in an airtight container and stored at room temperature up to 2 days.

Exchanges: 1 Carbohydrate • 1/2 Fat
Calories 98, Calories from Fat 26, Total Fat 3 g, Saturated Fat 1 g, Cholesterol 10 mg, Sodium 83 mg, Total Carbohydrate 17 g, Dietary Fiber 1 g, Sugars 8 g, Protein 2 g.

FLOURLESS PEANUT BUTTER COOKIES

Makes 20 servings • Serving size: 2 (1 3/4-inch) cookies

With a little less sugar and the substitution of natural peanut butter for the sweetened variety, these cookies offer a healthier version of an old-fashioned favorite.

1 cup creamy or chunky natural peanut butter

3/4 cup light brown sugar

1 large egg

1/4 teaspoon salt

1. Preheat the oven to 350°F. Line baking sheets with parchment paper and set aside.

2. Combine all the ingredients in a medium bowl and stir until the dough is smooth. Roll the dough into 40 balls, each about 2 teaspoons, and place on the prepared baking sheets about 1 1/2 inches apart. (Leave the dough in balls for a chewy, moist cookie, or press each one flat with the bottom of a glass dipped in flour for a crisp cookie.) Bake 10 to 12 minutes or until the bottoms of the cookies are lightly browned but the centers remain soft.

3. Cool the cookies on the baking sheets on wire racks for 2 minutes. Remove from the baking sheets and cool completely on the wire racks. The cookies can be covered in an airtight container and stored at room temperature up to 2 days.

Exchanges: 1 Carbohydrate • 1 Fat
Calories 116, Calories from Fat 60, Total Fat 7 g, Saturated Fat 1 g, Cholesterol 11 mg, Sodium 84 mg, Total Carbohydrate 11 g, Dietary Fiber 1 g, Sugars 8 g, Protein 4 g.

SUGAR COOKIE CUTOUTS

Makes 24 servings • Serving size: 2 (2-inch) cookies

When the kids want to get out the cookie cutters, this is the recipe to use. Rolling the dough out at room temperature and then chilling it makes the shapes easy to cut out—even for the littlest hands. Try the spice cookie variation using a gingerbread man cookie cutter.

2 cups all-purpose flour

1/2 teaspoon baking powder

1/4 teaspoon salt

3/4 cup granulated sugar

2/3 cup 67% vegetable oil butter-flavored spread, at room temperature

2 egg yolks

2 teaspoons vanilla extract

1. Combine the flour, baking powder, and salt in a medium bowl and whisk to mix well. Set aside.

2. Combine the sugar and butter-flavored spread in a large bowl and beat at medium speed until the mixture is fluffy. Beat in the egg yolks and vanilla. Add the flour mixture and beat at low speed until a stiff dough forms.

3. Divide the dough into two portions. Place each portion on a sheet of waxed paper and pat into rectangles. Top each portion of dough with waxed paper and roll to 1/8-inch thickness. Place the dough portions on a baking sheet and refrigerate 1 hour.

4. Preheat the oven to 350°F. Line baking sheets with parchment paper and set aside.

5. Working with one piece of dough at a time, remove the top sheet of waxed paper and cut the dough into desired shapes using 2-inch cookie cutters. Reroll the dough scraps and continue cutting out the cookies until all the dough is used. If the dough softens too much to cut out shapes easily, transfer the dough to the refrigerator and chill again. Place the cookies 1 inch apart on prepared baking sheets. Bake until the edges are lightly browned, 12 to 14 minutes.

6. Cool the cookies on the baking sheets on wire racks for 2 minutes. Remove from the baking sheets and cool completely on the wire racks. The cookies can be covered in an airtight container and stored at room temperature up to 3 days.

Variation

To make Spice Cookie Cutouts, add 2 teaspoons ground ginger, 1 teaspoon ground cinnamon, 1/2 teaspoon ground nutmeg, and 1/4 teaspoon ground cloves to the flour mixture.

Exchanges: 1 Carbohydrate • 1 Fat
Calories 106, Calories from Fat 42, Total Fat 5 g, Saturated Fat 1 g, Cholesterol 18 mg, Sodium 73 mg, Total Carbohydrate 14 g, Dietary Fiber 0 g, Sugars 6 g, Protein 1 g.

Sugar Drop Cookies

Makes 24 servings • Serving size: 2 (2-inch) cookies

Sometimes simplest is best. These homey, easy-to-make cookies are crispy on the edges and chewy on the inside—just right with a hot cup of tea.

2 cups all-purpose flour

1 tablespoon cornstarch

1/2 teaspoon baking soda

1/4 teaspoon salt

1/2 cup 67% vegetable oil butter-flavored spread, at room temperature

1/2 cup canola oil

3/4 cup plus 1 tablespoon granulated sugar, divided use

1 large egg

1 tablespoon vanilla extract

1. Combine the flour, cornstarch, baking soda, and salt in a medium bowl and whisk to mix well. Set aside.

2. Combine the butter-flavored spread and oil in a large bowl and beat at medium speed 2 minutes or until the mixture is smooth. Gradually beat in 3/4 cup of the sugar, beating until mixture is fluffy. Beat in the egg and vanilla. Add the flour mixture and beat at low speed until a stiff dough forms. Cover the dough and refrigerate 1 hour.

3. Preheat the oven to 350°F. Line baking sheets with parchment paper and set aside.

4. Roll the dough into 48 balls, 2 level teaspoons each, and place 2 inches apart on the prepared baking sheets. Flatten each ball with your fingers or make a crisscross design using a fork. Sprinkle the tops of cookies evenly with the remaining 1 tablespoon sugar. Bake until the edges are lightly browned, 10 to 12 minutes.

5. Cool the cookies on the baking sheets on wire racks for 2 minutes. Remove from the baking sheets and cool completely on the wire racks. The cookies can be covered in an airtight container and stored at room temperature up to 3 days.

Exchanges: 1 Carbohydrate • 1 1/2 Fat
Calories 138, Calories from Fat 72, Total Fat 8 g, Saturated Fat 1 g, Cholesterol 9 mg, Sodium 84 mg, Total Carbohydrate 15 g, Dietary Fiber 0 g, Sugars 7 g, Protein 1 g.

PISTACHIO ICEBOX COOKIES

Makes 48 servings • Serving size: 2 (1-inch) cookies

Keep a roll of these in the freezer at all times! They actually slice best
when frozen, so there's no waiting for the dough to defrost.

3/4 cup unsalted
pistachio nuts

2 cups all-purpose flour

1/2 teaspoon baking soda

1/4 teaspoon salt

1/2 cup 67% vegetable oil
butter-flavored spread, at
room temperature

1/4 cup canola oil

1 cup granulated sugar

2 egg yolks

2 teaspoons vanilla extract

1. Place the nuts in a food processor and process until finely chopped, but not ground. Set aside.

2. Combine the flour, baking soda, and salt in a medium bowl and whisk to mix well. Set aside.

3. Combine the butter-flavored spread and oil in a large bowl and beat at medium speed until mixture is smooth. Gradually beat in the sugar, beating until the mixture is fluffy. Beat in the egg yolks one at a time. Beat in the vanilla. Add the flour mixture and pistachios and beat at low speed until a stiff dough forms.

4. Divide the dough into 4 portions. Place each portion on a sheet of waxed paper and shape into a 6-inch log 1 inch in diameter. Wrap in plastic wrap and freeze 4 hours or up to 3 months.

5. Preheat the oven to 350°F. Line baking sheets with parchment paper and set aside.

6. Slice each log into 24 (1/4-inch) slices. Place on prepared baking sheets 1 inch apart and bake until the edges are lightly browned, 10 to 12 minutes.

7. Cool the cookies on the baking sheets on wire racks for 2 minutes. Remove from the baking sheets and cool completely on the wire racks. The cookies can be covered in an airtight container and stored at room temperature up to 3 days.

Exchanges: 1/2 Carbohydrate • 1 Fat
Calories 73, Calories from Fat 35, Total Fat 4 g, Saturated Fat 1 g, Cholesterol 9 mg, Sodium 41 mg, Total Carbohydrate 9 g, Dietary Fiber 0 g, Sugars 4 g, Protein 1 g.

MOLASSES SPICE DOMES

Makes 30 servings • Serving size: 2 (1 1/2-inch) cookies

These soft, cakey, spice-infused cookies aren't
beauty contest winners, but they're heavenly to eat!

2 1/2 cups all-purpose flour

2 teaspoons ground ginger

2 teaspoons ground cinnamon

1/2 teaspoon ground nutmeg

1/2 teaspoon ground cloves

1/2 teaspoon baking soda

1/4 teaspoon salt

1/2 cup canola oil

1/4 cup molasses

1/2 cup granulated sugar

2 large eggs

1 teaspoon vanilla extract

1. Combine the flour, ginger, cinnamon, nutmeg, cloves, baking soda, and salt in a medium bowl and whisk to mix well. Set aside.

2. Combine the oil, molasses, and sugar in a large bowl and beat at medium speed until mixture is smooth. Beat in the eggs one at a time. Beat in the vanilla. Add the flour mixture and beat at low speed until a stiff dough forms. Cover the dough and refrigerate 2 hours.

3. Preheat the oven to 350°F. Line baking sheets with parchment paper and set aside.

4. Roll the dough into 60 balls, 2 level teaspoons each, and place 2 inches apart on the prepared baking sheets. (For thinner cookies, moisten your fingertips with water and gently flatten each mound of dough.) Bake 8 to 10 minutes or until the bottoms of the cookies are lightly browned but the centers remain soft.

5. Cool the cookies on the baking sheets on wire racks for 2 minutes. Remove from the baking sheets and cool completely on the wire racks. The cookies can be covered in an airtight container and stored at room temperature up to 3 days.

Exchanges: 1 Carbohydrate • 1/2 Fat
Calories 96, Calories from Fat 37, Total Fat 4 g, Saturated Fat 1 g, Cholesterol 14 mg, Sodium 46 mg, Total Carbohydrate 13 g, Dietary Fiber 0 g, Sugars 5 g, Protein 2 g.

CHOCOLATE CRACKLES

Makes 26 servings • Serving size: 2 (1 1/2-inch) cookies

A plate of these little half moon cookies will put a smile on any face.
As the cookies bake, they expand, creating crackles in the sugar coating.

1 1/2 cups all-purpose flour

3/4 cup unsweetened cocoa

1 1/2 teaspoons
baking powder

1/4 teaspoon salt

1/2 cup 67% vegetable oil
butter-flavored spread, at
room temperature

1 cup dark brown sugar

2 large eggs

2 teaspoons vanilla extract

3 tablespoons
confectioners' sugar

1. Preheat the oven to 350°F. Line the baking sheets with parchment paper and set aside.

2. Combine the flour, cocoa, baking powder, and salt in a medium bowl and whisk to mix well. Set aside.

3. Combine the butter-flavored spread and brown sugar in a large bowl and beat at medium speed until mixture is fluffy. Beat in the eggs, one at a time. Beat in the vanilla. Add the flour mixture and beat at low speed until a stiff dough forms.

4. Place the confectioners' sugar in a shallow dish. Roll the dough into 52 balls, 2 level teaspoons each. Toss in confectioners' sugar to coat, shaking off excess. Place 1 inch apart on prepared baking sheets. Bake 8 to 10 minutes, or until cookies are lightly browned on the bottoms and have a crackled appearance on top.

5. Cool the cookies on the baking sheets on wire racks for 2 minutes. Remove from the baking sheets and cool completely on the wire racks. The cookies can be covered in an airtight container and stored at room temperature up to 3 days.

Exchanges: 1 Carbohydrate • 1/2 Fat
Calories 100, Calories from Fat 33, Total Fat 4 g, Saturated Fat 1 g, Cholesterol 16 mg, Sodium 81 mg, Total Carbohydrate 16 g, Dietary Fiber 1 g, Sugars 9 g, Protein 2 g.

ALMOND BUTTONS

Makes 16 servings • Serving size: 2 (1 1/2-inch) cookies

Crisp on the outside and chewy on the inside, this version of almond macaroons
is one of the easiest and most pleasing cookies you'll ever taste.

1/2 cup granulated sugar

1/4 cup all-purpose flour

1/4 teaspoon salt

7 ounces almond paste, crumbled

2 egg whites, at room temperature

32 whole blanched almonds

1. Preheat the oven to 350°F. Line two baking sheets with parchment paper and set aside.

2. Combine the sugar, flour, and salt in a medium bowl and whisk to mix well. Set aside.

3. Combine the almond paste and egg whites in a large bowl and beat at medium speed, about 3 minutes, or until mixture is smooth. Gradually beat in the sugar mixture.

4. Drop mounds of dough, about 2 teaspoons each, 1 inch apart, onto the prepared baking sheets. Gently press an almond into each cookie. Bake 12 to 14 minutes or until the edges of cookies are lightly browned.

5. Cool the cookies on the baking sheets on wire racks for 2 minutes. Remove from the baking sheets and cool completely on the wire racks. The cookies can be covered in an airtight container and stored at room temperature up to 4 days.

Exchanges: 1 Carbohydrate • 1 Fat
Calories 106, Calories from Fat 44, Total Fat 5 g, Saturated Fat 0 g, Cholesterol 0 mg, Sodium 44 mg, Total Carbohydrate 14 g, Dietary Fiber 1 g, Sugars 11 g, Protein 2 g.

PECAN CHEWS

Makes 12 servings • Serving size: 2 (2-inch) cookies

For nut lovers only, these delicate cookies are chewy in the center
and crisp on the edges. The texture softens when they're stored,
but they taste just as good. Try making them with walnuts, too.

1 cup pecan pieces

1/2 cup dark brown sugar

**2 tablespoons
all-purpose flour**

Pinch of salt

1 large egg

1. Preheat the oven to 350°F. Line the baking sheets with parchment paper and set aside.

2. Combine the pecans, brown sugar, flour, and salt in a food processor and pulse until the pecans are coarsely chopped. Add the egg and pulse until a stiff dough forms.

3. Drop mounds of dough, 2 level teaspoons each, 2 inches apart, onto the prepared baking sheets. Bake 10 to 12 minutes or until the cookies are lightly browned around the edges.

4. Cool the cookies on the baking sheets on wire racks for 2 minutes. Remove from the baking sheets and cool completely on the wire racks. The cookies can be covered in an airtight container and stored at room temperature up to 2 days.

Exchanges: 1 Carbohydrate • 1 Fat
Calories 110, Calories from Fat 65, Total Fat 7 g, Saturated Fat 1 g, Cholesterol 18 mg, Sodium 22 mg, Total Carbohydrate 11 g, Dietary Fiber 1 g, Sugars 9 g, Protein 2 g.

LEMONY OAT DROPS

Makes 20 servings • Serving size: 2 (1 1/2-inch) cookies

Don't panic when see how thin this dough is. It holds together just enough to bake up into moist, chewy cookies with a zing of citrus. And one teaspoon of flour is just enough!

1 1/2 cups quick-cooking oats

1/2 cup 67% vegetable oil butter-flavored spread, melted and cooled

3/4 cup granulated sugar

1 teaspoon all-purpose flour

1 teaspoon baking powder

1/4 teaspoon salt

1 large egg, lightly beaten

1/2 cup sliced almonds

1 tablespoon fresh grated lemon zest

1 teaspoon vanilla extract

1. Preheat the oven to 325°F. Line baking sheets with parchment paper and set aside.

2. Combine the oats and butter-flavored spread in a large bowl and stir to mix well. Add the remaining ingredients and stir until moistened.

3. Drop mounds of dough, 2 level teaspoons each, 2 inches apart, onto prepared baking sheets. Bake 10 to 12 minutes or until the edges of the cookies are lightly browned.

4. Cool the cookies on the baking sheets on wire racks for 2 minutes. Remove from the baking sheets and cool completely on the wire racks. The cookies can be covered in an airtight container and stored at room temperature up to 2 days.

Exchanges: 1 Carbohydrate • 1 Fat
Calories 104, Calories from Fat 49, Total Fat 5 g, Saturated Fat 1 g, Cholesterol 11 mg, Sodium 87 mg, Total Carbohydrate 12 g, Dietary Fiber 1 g, Sugars 8 g, Protein 2 g.

Spiced Date Softies

Makes 30 servings • Serving size: 2 (1 1/2-inch) cookies

To guarantee that the cookies turn out moist, make sure your dates haven't been stored too long. They should be supple and plump with no crystallized sugar on the outside.

2 1/2 cups all-purpose flour

2 teaspoons baking powder

1 teaspoon ground cinnamon

1/2 teaspoon baking soda

1/2 teaspoon ground allspice

1/4 teaspoon salt

1/4 teaspoon ground cloves

1/2 cup 67% vegetable oil butter-flavored spread, at room temperature

3/4 cup granulated sugar

1 large egg

1/2 cup 1% low-fat milk

1 teaspoon vanilla extract

1 cup pitted dates, coarsely chopped

1. Preheat the oven to 350°F. Line baking sheets with parchment paper and set aside.

2. Combine the flour, baking powder, cinnamon, baking soda, allspice, salt, and cloves in a medium bowl and whisk to mix well. Set aside.

3. Combine the butter-flavored spread and sugar in a large bowl and beat at medium speed until mixture is fluffy. Beat in the egg and milk. Beat in the vanilla. Add the flour mixture and beat at low speed until a stiff dough forms. Stir in the dates.

4. Roll the dough into 60 balls, 2 level teaspoons each, and place 2 inches apart on the prepared baking sheets. (For thinner cookies, moisten your fingertips with water and gently flatten each mound of dough.) Bake 10 to 12 minutes or until the bottoms of the cookies are lightly browned.

5. Cool the cookies on the baking sheets on wire racks for 2 minutes. Remove from the baking sheets and cool completely on the wire racks. The cookies can be covered in an airtight container and stored at room temperature up to 3 days.

Exchanges: 1 Carbohydrate • 1/2 Fat
Calories 101, Calories from Fat 26, Total Fat 3 g, Saturated Fat 1 g, Cholesterol 7 mg, Sodium 94 mg, Total Carbohydrate 18 g, Dietary Fiber 1 g, Sugars 9 g, Protein 2 g.

ALMOND BISCOTTI

Makes 16 servings • Serving size: 2 (1/2-inch) biscotti

These crunchy cookies turn afternoon coffee or tea break into something special.
They keep well, too—perfect to have on hand for an impromptu coffee klatch.

1/2 cup slivered almonds	3/4 cup granular no-calorie sweetener
2 cups all-purpose flour	1/2 cup granulated sugar
1 teaspoon baking powder	2 large eggs
1/2 teaspoon baking soda	1/4 cup 1% low-fat milk
1/8 teaspoon salt	1/4 teaspoon almond extract

1. Preheat the oven to 350°F. Coat a baking sheet with cooking spray and set aside.

2. Place the almonds in a small baking pan and bake 6 to 8 minutes, stirring once, or until lightly toasted. Set aside to cool. Maintain the oven temperature.

3. Combine the flour, baking powder, baking soda, and salt in a medium bowl and whisk to mix well. Set aside.

4. Combine the no-calorie sweetener, sugar, eggs, and milk in a large mixing bowl and beat at medium speed until the mixture is smooth. Beat in the almond extract. Add the flour mixture and beat at low speed until a stiff dough forms. Stir in the almonds.

5. Turn the dough out onto a lightly floured surface, sprinkle top of dough lightly with flour, and knead 6 to 8 times. Divide the dough in half and shape each portion into an 8-inch log. Place the logs on the prepared baking sheet and flatten slightly.

6. Bake 20 minutes or until the tops are firm to the touch and the bottoms are lightly browned. Maintain the oven temperature. Place the logs on a wire rack to cool for 20 minutes. Cut each log diagonally into 1/2-inch slices using a serrated knife. Place the slices on a parchment-lined baking sheet. Bake 8 minutes. Turn the biscotti over and bake 8 more minutes or until lightly browned. Place on wire racks to cool. The cookies can be covered in an airtight container and stored at room temperature up to 4 days.

Variation

To make Chocolate-Almond Biscotti, reduce the flour to 1 3/4 cup and add 1/3 cup unsweetened cocoa.

Exchanges: 1 1/2 Carbohydrate • 1/2 Fat
Calories 118, Calories from Fat 24, Total Fat 3 g, Saturated Fat 0 g, Cholesterol 27 mg, Sodium 92 mg, Total Carbohydrate 20 g, Dietary Fiber 1 g, Sugars 8 g, Protein 3 g.

Nutty Fruitcake Bites

Makes 25 servings • Serving size: 2 (1 1/2-inch) cookies

These are a fruitcake lover's dream. There's just enough of the spicy dough to hold the generous portion of fruit and nuts together.

3/4 cup all-purpose flour

1/2 teaspoon ground allspice

1/2 teaspoon ground cinnamon

1/2 teaspoon ground cloves

1/2 teaspoon baking soda

1/4 teaspoon salt

1/4 cup 67% vegetable oil butter-flavored spread, at room temperature

1/3 cup light brown sugar

1 large egg

2 teaspoons vanilla extract

3/4 cup chopped pecans or walnuts

3/4 cup pitted dates, chopped

1/2 cup dried apricots, chopped

1/4 cup golden raisins

1/4 cup dried currants

1. Preheat the oven to 350°F. Line baking sheets with parchment paper and set aside.

2. Combine the flour, allspice, cinnamon, cloves, baking soda, and salt in a medium bowl and whisk to mix well. Set aside.

3. Combine the butter-flavored spread and brown sugar in a large bowl and beat at medium speed until mixture is fluffy. Beat in the egg and vanilla. Add the flour mixture and beat at low speed until a stiff dough forms. Stir in the pecans, dates, apricots, raisins, and currants.

4. Drop mounds of dough, 2 level teaspoons each, 2 inches apart, on the prepared baking sheets. Bake until the bottoms of cookies are lightly browned but the centers remain soft, 8 to 10 minutes.

5. Cool the cookies on the baking sheets on wire racks for 2 minutes. Remove from the baking sheets and cool completely on the wire racks. The cookies can be covered in an airtight container and stored at room temperature up to 2 days.

Exchanges: 1 Carbohydrate • 1/2 Fat
Calories 97, Calories from Fat 38, Total Fat 4 g, Saturated Fat 1 g, Cholesterol 8 mg, Sodium 68 mg, Total Carbohydrate 15 g, Dietary Fiber 1 g, Sugars 10 g, Protein 1 g.

COCOA BROWNIES

Makes 16 servings • Serving size: 1 (2-inch) brownie

Rich, moist, and fudgy, these brownies are a real indulgence.

1/2 cup unsweetened cocoa

1/3 cup all-purpose flour

1/2 teaspoon baking powder

1/4 teaspoon salt

1/3 cup 67% vegetable oil butter-flavored spread, at room temperature

1 cup granulated sugar

2 large eggs

1 teaspoon vanilla extract

1. Preheat the oven to 350°F. Coat an 8 × 8-inch baking pan with cooking spray and set aside.

2. Combine the cocoa, flour, baking powder, and salt in a small bowl and whisk to mix well. Set aside.

3. Place the butter-flavored spread in a medium bowl and beat at medium speed until fluffy. Gradually beat in the sugar. Beat in the eggs, one at a time. Beat in the vanilla. Add the cocoa mixture and beat at low speed until moistened.

4. Spoon the batter into the prepared pan, smooth the top, and bake for 20 to 25 minutes or until a wooden toothpick inserted in the center of the brownies comes out clean.

5. Cool completely in the pan on a wire rack. Cut into 16 (2 × 2-inch) bars. The brownies can be covered in an airtight container and stored at room temperature up to 3 days.

Exchanges: 1 Carbohydrate • 1/2 Fat
Calories 102, Calories from Fat 37, Total Fat 4 g, Saturated Fat 1 g, Cholesterol 26 mg, Sodium 87 mg, Total Carbohydrate 16 g, Dietary Fiber 1 g, Sugars 13 g, Protein 2 g.

Raspberry–Almond Bars

Makes 16 servings • Serving size: 1 (2-inch) bar

Tangy raspberry preserves top a rich-tasting almond shortbread crust.
Make these with your favorite flavor of fruit preserves for variety.

1 1/2 cups all-purpose flour

1/3 cup confectioners' sugar

3/4 teaspoon baking soda

1/4 teaspoon salt

1/3 cup plus 2 tablespoons 67% vegetable oil butter-flavored spread, at room temperature

1 tablespoon canola oil

1/2 teaspoon almond extract

3/4 cup sugar-free red raspberry preserves

1/2 cup sliced almonds

1. Preheat the oven to 375°F. Line an 8 × 8-inch baking pan with aluminum foil, leaving a 3-inch overhang on two opposite sides. Coat the foil with cooking spray and set aside.

2. Combine the flour, confectioners' sugar, baking soda, and salt in a medium bowl and whisk to mix well. Set aside.

3. Place the butter-flavored spread, oil, and almond extract in a medium bowl and beat at medium speed until fluffy. Add the flour mixture and beat at low speed until a crumbly dough forms. Press the dough into bottom and 1/4 inch up the sides of the prepared pan. Spread the preserves evenly over the crust and sprinkle the almonds evenly over the preserves. Bake 20 to 25 minutes or until the edges are very lightly browned.

4. Cool in the pan on a wire rack. Lift from the pan using the overhanging foil and cut into 16 (2 × 2-inch) bars. The bars are best on the day they are made.

Exchanges: 1 Carbohydrate • 1 Fat
Calories 120, Calories from Fat 65, Total Fat 7 g, Saturated Fat 1 g, Cholesterol 0 mg, Sodium 135 mg, Total Carbohydrate 14 g, Dietary Fiber 1 g, Sugars 3 g, Protein 2 g.

Layered Oatmeal–Fig Bars

Makes 16 servings • Serving size: 1 (2-inch) bar

Once you've tried this heartier and tastier version of fig newtons,
you'll never go back to the store-bought ones.

8 ounces dried figs (about 10 figs), stemmed and chopped

1 cup orange juice

1 1/2 cups all-purpose flour

1 cup quick-cooking oats

2/3 cup light brown sugar

1/2 teaspoon ground cinnamon

1/4 teaspoon salt

1/2 cup canola oil

1 large egg

1. Preheat the oven to 350°F. Coat an 8 × 8-inch baking pan with cooking spray and set aside.

2. Combine the figs and the orange juice in a medium saucepan and bring to a boil. Reduce the heat, cover, and simmer, stirring occasionally, 15 to 20 minutes or until the figs are very tender and most of liquid is absorbed. Cool the fig mixture, place in a food processor, and puree.

3. Combine the flour, oats, brown sugar, cinnamon, and salt in a food processor and process until the oats are finely ground. Add the oil and egg and pulse until well combined. Press half of the flour mixture in the bottom of the prepared pan. Spread the fig mixture evenly over the flour mixture and top with the remaining flour mixture, pressing gently into the fig layer. Bake for 25 to 30 minutes or until very lightly browed on the edges.

4. Cool in the pan on a wire rack. Cut into 16 (2 × 2-inch) bars. The bars can be covered in an airtight container and stored at room temperature up to 1 day.

Exchanges: 2 Carbohydrate • 1 1/2 Fat
Calories 204, Calories from Fat 69, Total Fat 8 g, Saturated Fat 1 g, Cholesterol 13 mg, Sodium 46 mg, Total Carbohydrate 32 g, Dietary Fiber 2 g, Sugars 18 g, Protein 3 g.

Lemon Squares

Makes 16 servings • Serving size: 1 (2-inch) square

Tangy lemon filling tops a sweet shortbread base, making a perfect flavor combination. Dress these up with fresh berries for a dinner party dessert, or serve them plain for an afternoon treat.

Crust

1 1/2 cups all-purpose flour

1/3 cup confectioners' sugar

3/4 teaspoon baking soda

1/4 teaspoon salt

1/3 cup plus 2 tablespoons 67% vegetable oil butter-flavored spread, at room temperature

1 tablespoon canola oil

1 teaspoon vanilla extract

Filling

1 cup granular no-calorie sweetener

2 tablespoons all-purpose flour

1 cup fresh lemon juice

1 large egg

1 egg white

1 tablespoon fresh grated lemon zest

Make Crust

1. Preheat the oven to 350°F. Line an 8 × 8-inch baking pan with aluminum foil, leaving a 3-inch overhang on two opposite sides. Coat the foil with cooking spray and set pan aside.

2. Combine the flour, confectioners' sugar, baking soda, and salt in a medium bowl and whisk to mix well. Set aside.

3. Combine the butter-flavored spread and oil in a medium bowl and beat at medium speed until mixture is fluffy. Beat in the vanilla. Add the flour mixture and beat at low speed until a crumbly dough forms. Press the dough in the bottom and 1/4 inch up the sides of prepared pan. Bake 15 to 20 minutes or until crust is lightly browned.

Make Filling

1. Combine the no-calorie sweetener, flour, lemon juice, egg, egg white, and lemon zest in a medium bowl and whisk until smooth.

2. Remove the crust from oven and pour no-calorie sweetener mixture over the hot crust. Bake 15 to 20 minutes longer or until the filling is set.

3. Cool in the pan on a wire rack. Lift from the pan using the overhanging foil and cut into 16 (2 × 2-inch) bars. The bars can be covered in an airtight container and stored at room temperature up to 2 days.

Exchanges: 1 Carbohydrate • 1/2 Fat
Calories 110, Calories from Fat 55, Total Fat 6 g, Saturated Fat 1 g, Cholesterol 15 mg, Sodium 150 mg, Total Carbohydrate 12 g, Dietary Fiber 0 g, Sugars 2 g, Protein 2 g.

Pleasers from the Freezer

CHILLY CHOCOLATE, STRAWBERRY, AND VANILLA PIE

Makes 8 servings • Serving size: 1 slice with 1 tablespoon strawberry topping

Reminiscent of Neapolitan ice cream with its three distinctive flavors, this pie is as colorful as it is delicious.

9 chocolate graham crackers, crumbled (use 9 whole rectangles)

2 tablespoons 67% vegetable oil butter-flavored spread, melted and cooled

1 egg white

2 pints no-sugar-added fat-free vanilla ice cream, softened

8 tablespoons sugar-free strawberry ice cream topping

1. Preheat the oven to 350°F. Coat a 9-inch glass pie plate with cooking spray and set aside.

2. Place crumbled graham crackers in a food processor and process until finely ground. Transfer to a medium bowl and stir in the butter-flavored spread and egg white. Coat your hands lightly with cooking spray and press mixture into the bottom and up the sides of the prepared pie plate.

3. Bake 8 to 10 minutes or until the crust is lightly browned (small cracks may appear). Cool completely on a wire rack.

4. Place the ice cream in a large bowl, stirring until smooth. Spoon the ice cream into the center of the prepared crust. Working quickly and using an offset spatula, gently spread the ice cream mixture to the edges of the crust. Cover and freeze overnight. Drizzle each slice with 1 tablespoon strawberry topping.

Exchanges: 2 1/2 Carbohydrate
Calories 180, Calories from Fat 35, Total Fat 4 g, Saturated Fat 1 g, Cholesterol 5 mg, Sodium 235 mg, Total Carbohydrate 35 g, Dietary Fiber 6 g, Sugars 10 g, Protein 6 g.

FROZEN CHOCOLATE–PEANUT PIE

Makes 8 servings • Serving size: 1 slice with 1 tablespoon chocolate syrup

The peanut butter crust in this pie is a great way to make a little peanut butter go a long way. With the addition of chopped roasted peanuts in the ice cream, the peanutty flavor really comes through.

1/4 cup natural creamy peanut butter

2 tablespoons orange juice

9 low-fat graham crackers, crumbled (use 9 whole rectangles)

2 pints no-sugar-added fat-free chocolate ice cream, softened

1/4 cup chopped dry roasted peanuts

8 tablespoons sugar-free chocolate syrup

1. Coat a 9-inch glass pie plate with cooking spray and set aside.

2. Combine the peanut butter and orange juice in a medium bowl and whisk until smooth. Set aside. Place the crumbled graham crackers in a food processor and process until finely ground. Add the cracker crumbs to the peanut butter mixture, stirring until moistened. Coat your hands lightly with cooking spray and press the mixture into the bottom and up the sides of the prepared pie plate.

3. Place the ice cream in a large bowl, stirring until smooth. Stir in the peanuts. Spoon the ice cream mixture into the center of the prepared crust. Working quickly and using an offset spatula, gently spread the ice cream mixture to the edges of the crust. Cover and freeze overnight. Drizzle each slice with 1 tablespoon chocolate syrup.

Exchanges: 2 1/2 Carbohydrate • 1 Fat
Calories 228, Calories from Fat 67, Total Fat 7 g, Saturated Fat 1 g, Cholesterol 4 mg, Sodium 233 mg, Total Carbohydrate 37 g, Dietary Fiber 5 g, Sugars 13 g, Protein 8 g.

Frozen Strawberry Swirl Angel Pie

Makes 10 servings • Serving size: 1 slice

Try this recipe with other soft fruits such as peaches, mangos, or raspberries.
You only need about 1 cup of sliced fruit to flavor 3 cups of ice cream.
Garnish the pie with whatever fruit you use for the filling.

Crust

2 egg whites

1/4 teaspoon cream of tartar

1 teaspoon vanilla extract

1/4 cup granulated sugar

Filling

1 cup sliced strawberries

3 cups no-sugar-added fat-free
vanilla ice cream, softened

Garnish

Fresh whole strawberries
(optional)

Make Crust

1. Preheat the oven to 225°F. Coat a 9-inch glass pie plate with cooking spray and set aside.

2. Combine the egg whites and cream of tartar in a medium bowl and beat at medium speed until foamy. Beat in the vanilla. Gradually add the sugar and beat at high speed until stiff peaks form. Spread into the prepared pie plate, sloping the edges to form a shell. Bake 1 hour to 1 hour 15 minutes or until the meringue is dry. Cool in the pan on a wire rack.

Make Filling

1. Place the strawberries in a food processor and process until pureed.

2. Place the ice cream in a large bowl, stirring until smooth. Add the strawberry puree and gently swirl together without mixing completely. Spoon into the cooled meringue crust. Cover and freeze overnight.

3. Let stand at room temperature 10 minutes before slicing. Garnish with fresh strawberries, if desired.

Exchanges: 1 Carbohydrate
Calories 77, Calories from Fat 0, Total Fat 0 g, Saturated Fat 0 g, Cholesterol 2 mg, Sodium 53 mg, Total Carbohydrate 18 g, Dietary Fiber 3 g, Sugars 9 g, Protein 3 g.

LEMONADE FREEZER CAKE

Makes 24 servings • Serving size: 1 (3 × 1 1/2-inch) piece

Layers of lemon sorbet and vanilla ice cream make a sweet–tart topping for lemon cake.

2 cups cake flour

1 teaspoon baking powder

1 teaspoon baking soda

1/4 teaspoon salt

1/4 cup canola oil

1 large egg

1/3 cup granulated sugar

1/3 cup granular no-calorie sweetener

1 1/3 cups low-fat buttermilk

1 teaspoon lemon extract

1 tablespoon fresh grated lemon zest

2 cups lemon sorbet, softened

2 cups no-sugar-added fat-free vanilla ice cream, softened

1. Preheat the oven to 350°F. Coat a 13 × 9-inch baking pan with cooking spray and set aside.
2. Combine the flour, baking powder, baking soda, and salt in a medium bowl and whisk to mix well. Set aside.
3. Combine the oil and egg in a large bowl and beat at medium speed until well mixed. Gradually add the sugar and no-calorie sweetener and beat until the mixture is smooth. Add the flour mixture and the buttermilk alternately to the oil mixture, beginning and ending with the flour mixture, beating well after each addition. Beat in the lemon extract. Stir in the lemon zest.
4. Spoon the batter into the prepared pan, smooth the top, and bake for 15 to 18 minutes or until a wooden toothpick inserted in the center of the cake comes out clean. Cool the cake completely in the pan on a wire rack.
5. Place the sorbet in a medium bowl, stirring until smooth. Working quickly and using an offset spatula, spread the sorbet evenly over the cake layer. Cover and freeze 2 hours or until firm.
6. Place the ice cream in a medium bowl, stirring until smooth. Working quickly and using an offset spatula, spread ice cream evenly over sorbet. Cover and freeze overnight. Let the cake stand at room temperature 10 minutes before slicing.

Exchanges: 1 1/2 Carbohydrate

Calories 115, Calories from Fat 20, Total Fat 3 g, Saturated Fat 0 g, Cholesterol 10 mg, Sodium 125 mg, Total Carbohydrate 21 g, Dietary Fiber 1 g, Sugars 9 g, Protein 2 g.

CHOCOLATE–PEPPERMINT
ICE CREAM CAKE

Makes 16 servings • Serving size: 1 (2-inch) piece

Serve squares of this festive ice cream cake during the holidays,
or anytime you crave a perfect pairing of chocolate and mint.

3/4 cup all-purpose flour

1/2 cup unsweetened cocoa

3/4 teaspoon baking powder

1/4 teaspoon baking soda

1/4 teaspoon salt

1/2 cup granulated sugar

1/2 cup granular no-calorie sweetener

1/3 cup low-fat buttermilk

3 tablespoons canola oil

2 large eggs

3/4 teaspoon peppermint extract

1/2 teaspoon vanilla extract

2 pints no-sugar-added fat-free vanilla
ice cream, softened

8 sugar-free hard peppermint candies,
crushed (about 1/4 cup)

16 tablespoons sugar-free chocolate syrup

1. Preheat the oven to 350°F. Coat an 8 × 8-inch baking pan with cooking spray and set aside.

2. Combine the flour, cocoa, baking powder, baking soda, and salt in a medium bowl and whisk to mix well. Set aside.

3. Combine the sugar, no-calorie sweetener, buttermilk, oil, and eggs in a large bowl. Beat at medium speed for about 2 minutes or until the mixture is smooth and pale yellow in color. Beat in the peppermint and vanilla extracts. Add the flour mixture and beat at low speed just until blended.

4. Pour the batter into the prepared pan. Bake 15 minutes or until a wooden toothpick inserted in the center of the cake comes out clean. Cool in the pan on a wire rack for 10 minutes. Remove from the pan and cool completely on the wire rack.

5. Line an 8 × 8-inch baking pan with aluminum foil, leaving a 4-inch overhang on each side. Using a long serrated knife, cut the cake in half horizontally. Place the bottom layer of the cake in the prepared pan.

6. Place the ice cream in a large bowl, stirring until smooth. Stir in the candies. Working quickly and using an offset spatula, spread the ice cream mixture evenly over the cake. Place the top cake layer on the ice cream. Cover and freeze overnight. Drizzle each serving with 1 tablespoon chocolate syrup.

Exchanges: 2 Carbohydrate
Calories 142, Calories from Fat 33, Total Fat 4 g, Saturated Fat 1 g, Cholesterol 29 mg, Sodium 148 mg, Total Carbohydrate 27 g, Dietary Fiber 4 g, Sugars 12 g, Protein 4 g.

FROZEN ORANGE SOUFFLÉS

Makes 8 servings • Serving size: soufflé with 1/4 cup orange segments

Cool and refreshing, these soufflés are terrific to serve after a summer barbecue. They are completely make-ahead, and you can serve them with any seasonal fruit instead of the oranges.

2 cups fresh-squeezed orange juice

1/4 cup granulated sugar

1/4 cup granular no-calorie sweetener

1 large egg

3 tablespoons cornstarch

Pinch of salt

1 tablespoon fresh grated orange zest

1 cup cold fat-free milk

3 large navel oranges

1. Combine the orange juice, sugar, no-calorie sweetener, egg, cornstarch, and salt in a medium heavy-bottomed saucepan and whisk until smooth. Cook over medium heat, whisking constantly, about 6 minutes or until the mixture comes to a boil and thickens. Remove from the heat and stir in the orange zest. Transfer to a medium bowl and cover the surface with plastic wrap to prevent a skin from forming. Cool to room temperature.

2. Place the fat-free milk in a medium bowl and beat at high speed until tripled in volume and soft peaks form. Working quickly, fold the whipped fat-free milk into the orange juice mixture in three additions, mixing until no white streaks remain. Spoon mixture into 8 (6-ounce) custard cups. Cover and freeze overnight.

3. Cut a thin slice from the top and bottom of each of the oranges, exposing the flesh. Stand each orange upright, and using a sharp knife, thickly cut off the peel, following the contour of the fruit and removing all the white pith and membrane. Holding the orange over a medium bowl, carefully cut along both sides of each section to free it from the membrane. Discard any seeds and let the sections fall into the bowl.

4. To serve, run a thin knife around the edge of each soufflé and unmold onto shallow serving bowls. Arrange the orange segments evenly around each soufflé. Serve immediately.

Exchanges: 1 1/2 Carbohydrate
Calories 120, Calories from Fat 7, Total Fat 1 g, Saturated Fat 0 g, Cholesterol 27 mg, Sodium 44 mg, Total Carbohydrate 26 g, Dietary Fiber 2 g, Sugars 21 g, Protein 3 g.

Frozen Berry–Mango Bombe

Makes 16 servings • Serving size: 1 slice

This layered bombe makes a stunning presentation. Use your imagination and choose different sorbet or ice cream flavors for variety.

2 pints raspberry sorbet, softened

1 pint mango sorbet, softened

1 pint low-fat chocolate sorbet, softened

Fresh raspberries or sliced mango (optional)

1. Place a 2 to 2 1/2-quart mold or round-bottomed bowl in the freezer for 1 hour. Remove the mold or bowl from freezer and, if using a bowl, line it with plastic wrap, leaving a 4 inch overhang on the side.

2. Place the raspberry sorbet in a large bowl, stirring until smooth. Working quickly and using an offset spatula, spread sorbet evenly in the bottom and up the sides of the mold or bowl. Return to the freezer and freeze 1 hour or until firm.

3. Place the mango sorbet in a medium bowl, stirring until smooth. Working quickly and using an offset spatula, spread the mango sorbet evenly over the raspberry sorbet. Return to the freezer and freeze 1 hour or until firm.

4. Place the chocolate sorbet in a medium bowl, stirring until smooth. Working quickly and using an offset spatula, fill the remaining space with chocolate sorbet. Cover and freeze overnight.

5. To unmold from a mold, dip the mold into hot water for 30 seconds and invert the bombe onto a serving plate. To unmold from a bowl, uncover the bombe and use the overhanging plastic wrap to loosen from the sides of the bowl. Invert onto a serving plate and peel away the plastic wrap. Serve immediately, garnished with fresh berries or sliced mango, if desired.

Exchanges: 2 Carbohydrate

Calories 130, Calories from Fat 0, Total Fat 0 g, Saturated Fat 0 g, Cholesterol 0 mg, Sodium 20 mg, Total Carbohydrate 31 g, Dietary Fiber 2 g, Sugars 27 g, Protein 1 g.

RASPBERRY–VANILLA TERRINE

Makes 8 servings • Serving size: 1 (1-inch) slice with 1/2 tablespoon chocolate syrup

A "terrine" is a French word for an oval or rectangular cooking dish; it's also used to describe the food prepared in such a dish. Kids will love slices of this colorful treat as a summer refresher . . . or dress it up with a tumble of raspberries to appeal to adults.

2 pints no-sugar-added fat-free vanilla ice cream, softened, divided use

1 cup raspberry sorbet, softened

8 tablespoons sugar-free chocolate-flavored syrup

Fresh raspberries (optional)

1. Line an 8 × 4-inch loaf pan with foil, allowing the foil to extend over the edges of the pan. Place 1 pint of the ice cream in a medium bowl, stirring until smooth. Working quickly and using an offset spatula, spread the ice cream in the bottom of the pan. Freeze 1 hour or until firm.

2. Place the sorbet in a medium bowl, stirring until smooth. Working quickly and using an offset spatula, spread the sorbet evenly over the ice cream. Freeze 1 hour or until firm.

3. Place the remaining 1 pint of ice cream in a medium bowl, stirring until smooth. Working quickly and using an offset spatula, spread the ice cream over the sorbet. Cover the terrine with plastic wrap and freeze overnight.

4. Lift the terrine out of the pan using the foil overhang. To serve, place slices of the terrine on serving dishes and drizzle with chocolate syrup. Garnish with raspberries, if desired.

Exchanges: 2 Carbohydrate
Calories 117, Calories from Fat 0, Total Fat 0 g, Saturated Fat 0 g, Cholesterol 4 mg, Sodium 95 mg, Total Carbohydrate 30 g, Dietary Fiber 6 g, Sugars 14 g, Protein 4 g.

LAYERED ICE CREAM SQUARES

Makes 12 servings • Serving size: 1 (2 1/2 × 2-inch) piece

You can keep this dessert in the freezer for up to a week to serve at weeknight suppers or as a summer afternoon treat.

25 chocolate cookie wafers, crumbled

2 tablespoons 67% vegetable oil butter-flavored spread

1 egg white

2 pints no-sugar-added, fat-free vanilla ice cream, softened, divided use

1 pint no-sugar-added, fat-free chocolate ice cream, softened

12 tablespoons sugar-free chocolate syrup

1. Preheat the oven to 350°F. Coat an 8 × 8-inch baking pan with cooking spray and set aside.

2. Place the crumbled cookies in a food processor and process until finely ground. Transfer to a medium bowl and stir in the butter-flavored spread and egg white. Coat your hands lightly with cooking spray and press the mixture into the bottom of the prepared pan. Bake 8 minutes. Cool completely on a wire rack.

3. Place 1 pint of the vanilla ice cream in a medium bowl, stirring until smooth. Working quickly and using an offset spatula, gently spread the ice cream evenly over the crust. Freeze 1 hour or until firm. Place the chocolate ice cream in a medium bowl, stirring until smooth. Working quickly and using an offset spatula, gently spread the chocolate ice cream evenly over the vanilla ice cream. Freeze 1 hour or until firm. Place the remaining 1 pint of vanilla ice cream in a medium bowl, stirring until smooth. Working quickly and using an offset spatula, gently spread the vanilla ice cream over the chocolate ice cream.

4. Cover and freeze overnight. Let stand at room temperature for 5 minutes before slicing. Drizzle each serving with 1 tablespoon chocolate syrup.

Exchanges: 2 Carbohydrate • 1/2 Fat
Calories 160, Calories from Fat 31, Total Fat 3 g, Saturated Fat 1 g, Cholesterol 4 mg, Sodium 207 mg, Total Carbohydrate 32 g, Dietary Fiber 5 g, Sugars 11 g, Protein 5 g.

Frozen Lemon Tartlets

Makes 8 servings • Serving size: 1 tartlet

Serve these tartlets on their own, or deck them out for dinner with fresh berries
and the Vanilla Sauce on page 158. The sweet gingerbread crust is
just the right counterpoint to the tart lemon sorbet.

9 reduced-fat gingersnap cookies, crumbled

1 tablespoon 67% vegetable oil butter-flavored spread, melted and cooled

2 cups no-sugar-added lemon sorbet, softened

1. Line 8 muffin cups with paper liners.

2. Place the crumbled cookies in a food processor and process until finely ground. Transfer to a medium bowl and stir in the butter-flavored spread. Spoon about 1 tablespoon of the cookie mixture into each muffin cup and press into the bottom. Freeze 30 minutes.

3. Spoon 1/4 cup sorbet into each muffin cup, smoothing the tops. Freeze 4 hours or until firm. Allow to stand at room temperature 5 minutes before serving.

Exchanges: 1 1/2 Carbohydrate
Calories 95, Calories from Fat 20, Total Fat 2 g, Saturated Fat 1 g, Cholesterol 0 mg, Sodium 55 mg, Total Carbohydrate 19 g, Dietary Fiber 0 g, Sugars 16 g, Protein 0 g.

SUNSHINE SUNDAES

Makes 6 servings • Serving size: 1/4 cup ice cream with 1/4 cup fruit

With a jumble of sun-drenched tropical fruits, these sundaes will brighten any day. They're simple enough to be kid-friendly, yet delicious enough to serve to special guests.

1 tablespoon 67% vegetable oil butter-flavored spread

2 tablespoons light brown sugar

1 cup fresh pineapple cubes (1-inch cubes)

1/4 teaspoon ground cinnamon

1 small not-too-ripe banana, sliced

1/2 cup fresh mango cubes (1-inch cubes)

1 1/2 cups no-sugar-added fat-free vanilla ice cream

2 tablespoons sweetened flaked coconut, toasted

1. Melt the butter-flavored spread in a large nonstick skillet over medium heat. Add the brown sugar and pineapple and cook, stirring often, 5 minutes or until the pineapple is lightly browned. Stir in the cinnamon. Add the banana and mango and cook, stirring constantly, 1 to 2 minutes or until heated through.

2. To serve, scoop the ice cream into individual dessert bowls. Spoon the warm fruit mixture around the ice cream, dividing evenly. Sprinkle evenly with the coconut.

Exchanges: 1 1/2 Carbohydrate
Calories 115, Calories from Fat 20, Total Fat 2 g, Saturated Fat 1 g, Cholesterol 2 mg, Sodium 57 mg, Total Carbohydrate 25 g, Dietary Fiber 4 g, Sugars 14 g, Protein 2 g.

Cantaloupe Popsicles

Makes 6 servings • Serving size: 1 popsicle

Keep these on hand as a cool treat for kids of all ages. Try the popsicles with watermelon or honeydew cubes instead of cantaloupe, too.

3 cups fresh cantaloupe cubes (1-inch cubes)

2 tablespoons fresh lime juice

1. Combine the cantaloupe and lime juice in a food processor and process until smooth. Pour into 6 (2 1/2-ounce) freezer pop molds or into small paper cups.

2. Freeze 1 1/2 hours or until slushy. Insert popsicle sticks and freeze 6 hours or until firm. The popsicles will keep up to 1 week in the freezer.

Exchanges: 1/2 Fruit
Calories 29, Calories from Fat 0, Total Fat 0 g, Saturated Fat 0 g, Cholesterol 0 mg, Sodium 8 mg, Total Carbohydrate 7 g, Dietary Fiber 1 g, Sugars 6 g, Protein 1 g.

CRANBERRY–ORANGE SORBET

Makes 8 servings • Serving size: 1/4 cup sorbet with 1/4 cup orange segments

Guests will never guess the simple ingredients in this fancy-looking dessert.
It has the texture of soft-serve ice cream, but none of the fat.

**1 (16-ounce) can jellied
cranberry sauce**

**1 tablespoon fresh grated
orange zest**

**2 tablespoons fresh-squeezed
orange juice**

4 large navel oranges

1. Freeze the cranberry sauce in the can overnight.

2. Stand the unopened can under hot running water for 30 seconds. Spoon the cranberry sauce into a food processor, add orange zest and orange juice, and process 1 minute or until smooth. The sorbet may be served immediately or stored in the freezer in an airtight container up to 1 day.

3. Cut a thin slice from the top and bottom of each of the oranges, exposing the flesh. Stand each fruit upright, and using a sharp knife, thickly cut off the peel, following the contour of the fruit and removing all the white pith and membrane. Holding the fruit over a bowl, carefully cut along both sides of each section to free it from the membrane. Discard any seeds and let the sections fall into the bowl.

4. To serve, spoon the sorbet into individual dessert bowls. Spoon the orange segments around the sorbet, dividing evenly.

Exchanges: 2 Carbohydrate
Calories 131, Calories from Fat 0, Total Fat 0 g, Saturated Fat 0 g, Cholesterol 0 mg, Sodium 16 mg, Total Carbohydrate 33 g, Dietary Fiber 3 g, Sugars 30 g, Protein 1 g.

MANGO–GINGER SORBET

Makes: 4 servings • Serving size: 1/2 cup

You can't get a bigger punch of flavor with less effort than with this smashing sorbet. Be sure to use ripe mangos—they'll be yellow with a blush of red and will give slightly to gentle pressure—and you're in for a knock-your-socks-off treat.

1/4 cup water

1/4 cup granulated sugar

1/4 cup granular no-calorie sweetener

4 ripe mangos, peeled, pitted, and chopped (about 2 cups)

1 teaspoon fresh grated ginger

2 tablespoons fresh lime juice

1. Combine the water, sugar, and no-calorie sweetener in a small saucepan. Bring to a boil, stirring until sugar dissolves. Cool slightly.

2. Combine the sugar mixture, mangos, ginger, and lime juice in a food processor and process until smooth. Transfer to an airtight container and freeze overnight or until firm. Let stand at room temperature 15 minutes before serving.

Exchanges: 2 Carbohydrate
Calories 110, Calories from Fat 0, Total Fat 0 g, Saturated Fat 0 g, Cholesterol 0 mg, Sodium 3 mg, Total Carbohydrate 29 g, Dietary Fiber 2 g, Sugars 26 g, Protein 0 g.

REAL FROZEN YOGURT

Makes 12 servings • Serving size: 1/3 cup

This is genuine frozen yogurt—sweet and tangy all in one bite—and far better than what you buy at the supermarket. Try the stir-in options for an even more scrumptious dessert.

2 (32-ounce) containers plain low-fat yogurt

1/4 cup light corn syrup

1/4 cup granular no-calorie sweetener

2 teaspoons vanilla extract

1. Line a sieve or a colander with several thicknesses of cheesecloth and set over a bowl. Spoon the yogurt into the sieve, cover, and refrigerate overnight.

2. Combine the drained yogurt, corn syrup, no-calorie sweetener, and vanilla in a large bowl and whisk until smooth. Spoon into an ice cream maker and freeze according to manufacturer's instructions. Serve immediately for a soft-serve ice cream texture, or spoon into an airtight container and freeze overnight for firmer texture. Let stand at room temperature 10 minutes before serving.

Variations

AMARETTO CRUNCH: Stir in 1 cup crumbled biscotti and 2 tablespoons amaretto liqueur after freezing in the ice cream maker.

CHOCOLATE CHERRY: Stir in 1/4 cup grated bittersweet chocolate and 1 cup fresh pitted cherries after freezing in the ice cream maker.

PEACHY PECAN: Stir in 1 cup chopped fresh peaches and 1/3 cup toasted chopped pecans after freezing in the ice cream maker.

Exchanges: 1 Carbohydrate • 1/2 Fat
Calories 110, Calories from Fat 20, Total Fat 2 g, Saturated Fat 1 g, Cholesterol 10 mg, Sodium 95 mg, Total Carbohydrate 15 g, Dietary Fiber 0 g, Sugars 7 g, Protein 8g

Vanilla Ice Cream

Makes 6 servings • Serving size: 1/2 cup

This better-than-store-bought vanilla ice cream is a special treat on its own, and it makes an excellent starting point for all kinds of additions. Try the ideas below or invent your own.

2 cups 1% low-fat milk

2 large eggs

1/4 cup granulated sugar

1/4 cup granular no-calorie sweetener

Pinch of salt

1 teaspoon vanilla extract

1. Combine the milk, eggs, sugar, no-calorie sweetener, and salt in a medium heavy-bottomed saucepan and whisk until smooth. Cook over medium-low heat, whisking constantly, about 5 minutes or until mixture thickens slightly (do not allow to boil or mixture will curdle).

2. Transfer to a medium bowl and cool to room temperature. Stir in the vanilla. Cover and refrigerate 2 hours. Pour into an ice cream maker and freeze according to manufacturer's instructions. Serve at once for a soft-serve ice cream texture, or spoon into an airtight container and freeze overnight for firmer texture. Let stand at room temperature 10 minutes before serving.

Variations

CHOCOLATE: Add 1/4 cup unsweetened cocoa to the milk mixture before cooking.

STRAWBERRY: Stir 1 cup chopped fresh strawberries into the ice cream after freezing in the ice cream maker.

LEMON: Substitute 1 tablespoon fresh grated lemon zest for the vanilla.

PEPPERMINT: Substitute 1/2 teaspoon peppermint extract for the vanilla; garnish each serving with crushed sugar-free hard peppermint candies.

Exchanges: 1 Carbohydrate • 1/2 Fat
Calories 99, Calories from Fat 22, Total Fat 2 g, Saturated Fat 1 g, Cholesterol 76 mg, Sodium 89 mg, Total Carbohydrate 14 g, Dietary Fiber 0 g, Sugars 13 g, Protein 5 g.

Index

Tarts

OTHER TITLES FROM THE AMERICAN DIABETES ASSOCIATION

To order these and other great American Diabetes Association titles, call 1-800-232-6733 or visit *http://store.diabetes.org.* American Diabetes Association titles are also available in bookstores nationwide.

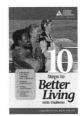

10 Steps to Better Living with Diabetes
by Ginger Kanzer-Lewis, RN, BC, EdM, CDE
Don't let diabetes take control of your life. Instead, take control of your diabetes! Learn the answers to all of your questions about self-care, including the questions you didn't even know to ask. Start living a better life with diabetes—let Ginger Kanzer-Lewis show you how.
Order no. 4882-01; Price $16.95

American Diabetes Association Complete Guide to Diabetes, 4th Edition
by American Diabetes Association
Have all the tips and information on diabetes that you need close at hand. The world's largest collection of diabetes self-care tips, techniques, and tricks for solving diabetes-related problems is back in its fourth edition, and it's bigger and better than ever before.
Order no. 4809-04; Price $29.95

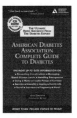

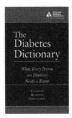

The Diabetes Dictionary
by American Diabetes Association
Diabetes can be a complicated disease; so to stay healthy, you need to understand the growing vocabulary of diabetes research and treatment. *The Diabetes Dictionary* gives straightforward definitions of diabetes terms and concepts that you need to manage your disease. With more than 500 entries, this is an indispensable resource for every person with diabetes.
Order no. 5020-01; Price $5.95

Diabetes Fit Food
by Ellen Haas
Put tasteless, boring recipes in the past with this new diabetes cookbook from healthy-eating expert Ellen Haas. She has compiled amazing, healthy recipes from some of America's best celebrity chefs, including Todd English, Alice Waters, and others. Finally, you can make sensible, healthy eating taste like it comes from a five-star restaurant.
Order no. 4661-01; Price $16.95

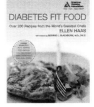

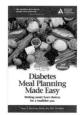

Diabetes Meal Planning Made Easy, 3rd Edition
by Hope S. Warshaw, MMSc, RD, CDE, BC-ADM

Let expert Hope Warshaw show you how to change unhealthy eating habits while continuing to enjoy the foods you love! This book serves up techniques for changing | your eating habits over time so that changes you make are the ones that last for life! Order no. 4706-03; Price $14.95

The "I Hate to Exercise" Book for People with Diabetes, 2nd Edition
by Charlotte Hayes, MMSc, MS, RD, CDE

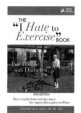

Get these "I hate to exercise" exercises and get-fit tricks for the uninitiated, unmotivated, and unlikely to exercise person with diabetes. If you hate to exercise and find it a chore or a challenge, this book is for you! Everyday activities can help you reap the benefits of exercise simply by using your arms more, bending your knees a little deeper, or putting more muscle behind it. Order no. 4837-02; Price $14.95

Holly Clegg's Trim & Terrific™ Diabetic Cooking
by Holly Clegg

Cookbook author Holly Clegg has teamed up with the American Diabetes Association to create a Trim & Terrific™ cookbook perfect for people with diabetes. With over 250 recipes, this collection is packed with meals that are quick, easy, and delicious. Forget the hassles of meal planning and rediscover the joys of great food! Order no. 4883-01; Price $18.95

The 4-Ingredient Diabetes Cookbook
by Nancy S. Hughes

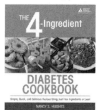

Making delicious meals doesn't have to be complicated, time-consuming, or expensive. You can create satisfying dishes using just four ingredients (or even fewer)! Make the most of your time and money. You'll be amazed at how much you can prepare with just a few simple ingredients. Order no. 4662-01; Price $16.95

To order these and other great American Diabetes Association titles, call 1-800-232-6733 or visit *http://store.diabetes.org.* American Diabetes Association titles are also available in bookstores nationwide.

About the American Diabetes Association

The American Diabetes Association is the nation's leading voluntary health organization supporting diabetes research, information, and advocacy. Its mission is to prevent and cure diabetes and to improve the lives of all people affected by diabetes. The American Diabetes Association is the leading publisher of comprehensive diabetes information. Its huge library of practical and authoritative books for people with diabetes covers every aspect of self-care—cooking and nutrition, fitness, weight control, medications, complications, emotional issues, and general self-care.

To order American Diabetes Association books: Call 1-800-232-6733 or log on to *http://store.diabetes.org*

To join the American Diabetes Association: Call 1-800-806-7801 or log on to *www.diabetes.org/membership*

For more information about diabetes or ADA programs and services: Call 1-800-342-2383. E-mail: AskADA@diabetes.org or log on to *www.diabetes.org*

To locate an ADA/NCQA Recognized Provider of quality diabetes care in your area: *www.ncqa.org/dprp*

To find an ADA Recognized Education Program in your area: Call 1-800-342-2383. *www.diabetes.org/for-health-professionals-and-scientists/recognition/edrecognition.jsp*

To join the fight to increase funding for diabetes research, end discrimination, and improve insurance coverage: Call 1-800-342-2383. *www.diabetes.org/advocacy-and-legalresources/advocacy.jsp*

To find out how you can get involved with the programs in your community: Call 1-800-342-2383. See below for program Web addresses.

American Diabetes Month: educational activities aimed at those diagnosed with diabetes—month of November. *www.diabetes.org/communityprograms-and-localevents/americandiabetesmonth.jsp*

American Diabetes Alert: annual public awareness campaign to find the undiagnosed—held the fourth Tuesday in March. *www.diabetes.org/communityprograms-and-localevents/americandiabetesalert.jsp*

American Diabetes Association Latino Initiative: diabetes awareness program targeted to the Latino community. *www.diabetes.org/communityprograms-and-localevents/latinos.jsp*

African American Program: diabetes awareness program targeted to the African American community. *www.diabetes.org/communityprograms-and-localevents/africanamericans.jsp*

Awakening the Spirit: Pathways to Diabetes Prevention & Control: diabetes awareness program targeted to the Native American community. *www.diabetes.org/communityprograms-and-localevents/nativeamericans.jsp*

To find out about an important research project regarding type 2 diabetes: *www.diabetes.org/diabetes-research/research-home.jsp*

To obtain information on making a planned gift or charitable bequest: Call 1-888-700-7029. *www.wpg.cc/stl/CDA/homepage/1,1006,509,00.html*

To make a donation or memorial contribution: Call 1-800-342-2383. *www.diabetes.org/support-the-cause/make-a-donation.jsp*